ENDURANCE

THE EVENTS, THE ATHLETES, THE ATTITUDE

Albert C. Gross

DODD, MEAD & COMPANY
New York

Dedicated to Cosette

Published by Dodd, Mead & Company, Inc.
79 Madison Avenue, New York, N.Y. 10016

Distributed in Canada by
McClelland and Stewart Limited, Toronto

Manufactured in the United States of America

Design and drawings by Jeremiah B. Lighter

First Edition

Library of Congress Cataloging-in-Publication Data

Gross, Albert C.
  Endurance: the events, the athletes, the attitude.

  Bibliography: p.
  Includes index.
  1. Endurance sports.   2. Physical education and
training.   3. Endurance sports—Psychological aspects.
I. Title.
GV749.5.G76   1986   796'.01   85-28062
ISBN 0-396-08393-5

1 2 3 4 5 6 7 8 9 10

CONTENTS

PART 5 THE LIMITS OF ENDURANCE

ACKNOWLEDGMENTS

I WISH to thank the numerous athletes who generously gave their time for interviews and permitted me to discuss their experiences. Similarly, I appreciate the candor and efforts of many race directors, event promoters, and officials of national sport federations.

I also wish to thank Terry Mulgannon and Harald Johnson at *Triathlon* magazine for providing answers to several research questions and helping me locate photos to illustrate the book. I am grateful to Cathy Hoy and the producers of the Bud Light United States Triathlon Series, who graciously provided numerous photographs for *Endurance*. Larry Cruse and other research librarians at the University of California, San Diego, deserve my gratitude for helping me answer many historical questions. My appreciation also goes to my friends John Newland, John Pappas, and John Howard, who commented on the manuscript, and to my friend Bob Arganbright, who helped me proofread the galleys.

Several colleagues researched and wrote the first versions of parts of the manuscript. Diane Thomas drafted Chapter 17 and Chapter 18. John Lehrer wrote the initial text for Chapter 9. Chapter 13 was drafted by Cheri Rae Wolpert. Patricia Hunt wrote the first avatar of Chapter 16's section on physiological limits. Christian Paul generously gave me permission to adapt part of Chapter 3's section on ride and ties and the description of hallucinations in Chapter 18 from manuscripts he wrote. Since I revised their work to reflect my own opinions and style preferences, I wish to absolve my colleagues of any responsibility for points of view expressed in the book. I remain indebted for their contributions, but I am responsible for any errors or shortcomings.

Ann Page and Eunice Heideman typed the manuscript, patiently coping with numerous revisions and tight deadlines. Perhaps more than anybody involved with this project, they understand the meaning of this book's title. They are *endurance* typists.

I am more indebted to Lois Krieger than most authors are to their editors. She responded to a proposal for a narrowly focused biography about a bicyclist by encouraging me to write *Endurance*. Then she called on her considerable skill as a professional editor and her personal background as an amateur triathlete to enhance that book.

INTRODUCTION

GRADUALLY, the radio penetrates Eric's sleeping consciousness. At first his somnolent mind is able to weave the instant-coffee commercial into a disjointed dream about a childhood ski holiday. Somehow he is skiing down a mountain of incongruously brown snow, whose flakes have the texture of instant-coffee grounds. Then the dream images become increasingly remote as he awakens. He begins to feel the slight muscle soreness and tightness of his right shoulder that have plagued him the past few months. The dream slips from his mind entirely when Marsha groans and pokes him in the ribs. Suddenly, completely awake, Eric automatically reaches for the button that will silence the cursed alarm radio. In the dark room the red numbers of the radio's digital display assault his bleary eyes to inform him that it is 4:30 A.M.

Slowly, Eric does a mental inventory of his body's physical condition. Not an ordinary body, but that of a thirty-eight-year-old endurance athlete. A body that has been developed, honed, and trained. A body that has been challenged, stretched, exerted, and sometimes overtrained. First the sore shoulder: "Well, a little better than Saturday; it will make it through the workout." Then the forearms and biceps: "No problem there; plenty of strength." Then the lower back: "A little rough, but OK," as he contemplates his abdominal muscles, which have been hardened like a washboard by thousands of sit-ups. Strong abdominals protect the lower back. Neck muscles: "No tightness. Good!"

Still wrapped in the blankets, Eric stretches his legs to work out the kinks in the joints of his lower limbs, a good stretch that makes his ankles crack, as he flattens his arches and points his toes toward the bedroom wall.

Eric turns to his wife, gives her a gentle kiss on the back of the neck, and raises his head slightly to whisper, "You go back to sleep. I've got to go down to the boathouse. I'll reset the alarm for you." In a groggy voice, Marsha responds, "Stay here, it's dark out there."

Eric lowers his head to the pillow in acquiescence. But then Marsha pokes him again. "Hey! You'd better get going. They'll be waiting for you."

Twenty years of devotion to rowing has instilled some discipline in Eric. Instantly he is out of the warm nest and into the cold bathroom to wash away the sleep and scrape the whiskers off his chin. Another few minutes and he has pulled on a warm sweatsuit and grabbed the bag of clean clothes he set out the night before. Then he is out the door. As he turns the key in the ignition of his car, Eric glances at his watch: 4:52. He might make it on time, if he can just avoid the red light at the bottom of the hill. No traffic to worry about at this hour.

At 5:17 he hears the reassuring sound of gravel beneath his wheels as he turns into the boathouse parking lot. Two minutes late, but he can already tell he isn't last. True to form, Fred is missing; he'll probably be along in another five minutes or so. Eric quickly grabs his gym bag, locks the car, and hurries to assist the rest of the crew, who are already carrying the oars and eight-man shell to the water.

Soon Fred also strides down to the dock. Another few minutes and the boat is rigged and launched with an eight-man crew and coxswain aboard. It is 5:30 A.M. Eastern Standard Time.

Meanwhile, two-thirds of a continent to the west, it is 3:30 A.M. Mountain Time. A motor home laboriously chugs up a steep hill at 10 miles per hour. The vehicle's lights cast eerie long shadows of a slowly churning lone cyclist, who is riding a few yards ahead. The cyclist flinches and is shaken from his weary, predawn reverie by an insect dive-bombing his head on its way to a collision with the motor home's right headlamp.

The driver of the motor home is fighting desperately to stay awake. On that dark and chill highway, with neither spectators nor other competitors in sight, it would be difficult to characterize the bizarre scene as an exciting moment in an athletic contest. Nonetheless, the bicyclist is a member of an elite group of competitive athletes who have qualified for the Race Across AMerica, the RAAM. And at 3:30 A.M. he is racing furiously to catch cyclists who are a hundred or more miles ahead. Several days earlier, amid much fanfare, he had left California's Santa Monica Pier. Before him stretches the remainder of the 3,047-mile road to the Atlantic City boardwalk. Along the way he will miss much sleep, and perhaps he will overtake one or more of the other riders.

As he rhythmically turns the cranks of his $1,500 racing machine, the cyclist's thoughts sink into a motivational abyss, which he usually tries to avoid. He muses, "*Why* am I doing this? I'm God knows how many hours behind the leader, I'm sleepy, and I ache all over. If I fall asleep, I'll be digging road grit out of my abrasions for days, and I'll probably trash my bike too. In the unlikely event that I catch up and reach the boardwalk first, all I'll win is $1,500. Nice of that bike shop to put that money up, but $1,500 is a pittance next to the thousands I've spent on this futile escapade. Let me see: there's food, gasoline, and the cost to rent the motor home. Crap, just think how much I spent for the qualifier, the John Marino Open . . ." Then, getting control of this dangerous train of thought: "Oh, what's the use? If I wanted to make money, I'd become a stockbroker or a real estate speculator. This is what I want to do. Who cares if I make money at this? Lon Haldeman's probably the only one making a living out of this, and he's not getting rich. Just keep pedaling. I'll take a nap in another couple of hours, and then I'll feel great."

His little morale crisis resolved, the lone cyclist pedals on into the early morning. On and on and on he pedals, a seemingly endless ribbon of highway ahead of him, for at least the next six or seven days and nights.

Another time zone to the west it is 2:30 A.M., and in Irvine, California, Tina Maria Stone is still fast asleep. In her dream she is running comfortably and steadily on a country road. When she awakens from her dream, Tina must suppress a temptation to run at 2:30 A.M. Tina goes back to sleep for another hour and a half. She will awaken naturally—before her alarm—and be out on the streets of Irvine by 4:30. At that hour she is still the only runner on the roads, and the local police protectively keep an eye out for her.

To say that Tina also runs during her waking hours would be an egregious understatement. Tina Maria Stone holds the record for the most miles run by any one human during one year. In 1983 she ran 15,472 miles. That distance, well over half the circumference of the earth, averages to 42.39 miles per day. Although she ran more miles on some of those days and fewer on others, she did in fact run on every single day of 1983. What's more, Stone claims that she never suffers running injuries. Tina stands five foot three and weighs a little less than 90 pounds. She has run several sub-three hour marathons. Since her record-setting year, Tina has decreased her running to "only" 25 to 30 miles per day.

Born in Naples, Italy, in 1934, Tina was only a few months shy of the half-century mark when she set her record. In fact, this ultra-distance runner can visit her two grandchildren when she runs near her daughter's house in El Toro. Running through the fragrant orange groves of El Toro reminds Tina of the country road in her recurring dream.

As a child Tina ran for transportation when her mother would

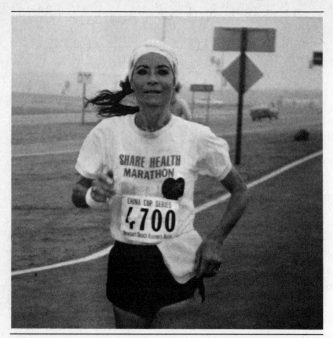

Tina Maria Stone, the undisputed mileage champion.
PHOTO BY ANNA CETO

send her on errands. Cars and bicycles were out of the question for Tina; her family suffered from the poverty of prewar Italy. Tina feels she was born to run, but she did not run as an adult until 1978.

Now, Tina Maria Stone lives to run. She believes she is addicted to running, and it would be difficult to refute her claim. But she sees her addiction in a positive light. She says, "Running is the greatest thing that ever happened to me. It keeps me sane. I take out my frustrations running. When I run, my mind gets totally lost until I'm done, and I look at the clock."

WHAT IS GOING ON?

Why are Eric and his teammates digging their oars into the still waters of an eastern river before going off to work? Why is a lone cyclist cranking along a mountain road at 3:30 in the morning? Why will Tina run 30 or more miles today, only to do the same thing tomorrow?

For modern society, mass participation in endurance athletics is a relatively recent phenomenon. It is speculated, however, that our ancient forebears were ultradistance runners, and there always have been aberrant individuals and groups who were endurance athletes; but only in the last fifteen years or so have large numbers of people adopted endurance sport as a way of life. That "phenomenon" may be of great social importance, and its meaning, character, and causes are well worth examining. Why is endurance sport blossoming in the last quarter of the twentieth century, as never before?

What is this endurance business all about? This book explores those questions.

The Events

The term "endurance" is used rather loosely in the vernacular to mean anything done for a long time. Thus, when Rena Clark and Jeff Block rode a Ferris wheel for thirty-seven continuous days, they set an endurance record of sorts. A record of that type is entertaining, but by and large it is best reserved for the *Guinness Book of Records*. In this book we will use the term "endurance event" only as it applies to athletics.

In general, the endurance sports covered here involve some form of human-powered locomotion. Sometimes the athletes proceed entirely under their own power, as would be the case for swimming, running, and racewalking. Other times endurance athletes must rely on equipment, such as bicycles, cross-country skis, rowing shells, kayaks, canoes, mountain-climbing gear, or even human-powered aircraft. Occasionally, an animal is a partner in the endurance endeavor, as in long-distance horseback riding and dog sledding.

In recent years a great deal of ingenuity has been expended concocting multisport events, which combine several of the traditional endurance sports to produce hybrids, such as bike-swim-run triathlons, run-bike biathlons, and ride and ties. (In a ride and tie two runners share one horse, taking turns riding and running.) Multisport events are different from their constituent parts, and this book covers them too.

To characterize an event as an example of endurance sport, however, more than mere locomotion is required. The territory of this book is long- and ultralong-distance events. The 60-yard dash is a fine contest, but this book will politely ignore any footrace shorter than a marathon. (In the world of ultradistance running, life begins at 26 miles.) Slalom and other Alpine skiing events are exhilarating spectacles, but the turf here is cross-country or Nordic skiing, with a special bias toward the longer events, such as the 55-kilometer Birkebeiner. For this book, swims longer than 2 miles and bike races longer than 100 miles would qualify as endurance events, although endurance swimmers and cyclists frequently exceed those distances by a great deal.

Part I of this book describes the events that constitute endurance sport.

The Endurance Athletes

Some rowers, cyclists, runners, and other athletes push their minds and bodies beyond conventional limits. Those athletes transcend physical fitness in order to challenge the very boundaries of physiological and mental endurance. They run the gamut of ability in their sports from world-class to ordinary performer. Yet even the humblest endurance athlete does some extraordinary things.

Some endurance athletes pursue their sports single-mindedly, with no other occupation or profession. For instance, Australian Joe Record, who ran 470 miles for a third-place finish in the 1983 New York Road Runners Club Six-Day Footrace, describes his occupation as "being a bum." He jokingly calls himself a "self-educated student of philosophy, psychology, and medicine." Record dabbles in odd jobs, such as house painting, to support his ultradistance running.

Ron Laird, a champion racewalker who won a gold medal in the 1967 Pan American Games, finances a Spartan existence on minuscule sponsorships. An athletic vagabond, Laird travels the world from one race or handout to another. He won sixty-five U.S. National titles in his sport between 1958 and 1976, and he represented the United States in four Olympiads. Although some countries—e.g., East Germany— provide sports sinecures to support the training of its athletes of comparable ability, in the United States, Laird, who practices an obscure amateur sport, has lived in poverty during his years of greatest competitive success. (Racewalkers, unlike runners, must have one foot on the ground at all times, and must lock one knee on each step.)

A tiny minority of professionals do make a comfortable living from endurance sport, though. In 1984, triathlete Scott Molina earned $51,000 in prize money. Bicycle road-race world champion Greg LeMond and marathoners such as Frank Shorter, Bill Rodgers, and Alberto Salazar all pull down six-figure incomes.

Still, most endurance athletes are amateurs, and many successfully practice other professions. Peter Penseyres, who bicycled to victory in the 1984 Race Across AMerica, is a nuclear engineer, employed full-time by Southern California Edison Power Company. Don Choi of San Francisco once ran 511.25 miles in six days and is considered the father of the modern six-day footrace, but running is merely his avocation; he carries a mail sack for the U.S. Postal Service, usually running his route.

Endurance athletes are amateur and professional, young and old, rich and poor, female and male. They come from all over the world. They practice many different sports. Some endurance athletes have overcome disabilities and physical handicaps, and often their accomplishments greatly surpass the prowess of so-called normal people.

In Part II of this book you will find information about the athletes who practice endurance sport.

Why?

The most frequently asked question about ultradistance sport is "Why do they do it?" Part III takes up that question fully. Part IV discusses how to find the endurance athlete in yourself. One question asked is "Do you need to be a champion?" Part IV also explores the world of the female endurance athlete and includes a how-to chapter on getting involved in endurance sport. Another chapter examines the effect of endurance sport on relationships.

Boundaries of Endurance

What are the limits of our endurance? Endurance sport is more than a casual commitment; for many it is a way of life. Sometimes endurance sport is a threat to life itself: on a few occasions endurance athletes have pushed themselves beyond the brink of death.

Records in sport seem to improve continuously. Is the human capacity for athletic improvement infinite? The last section of this book looks at the ultimate limits of endurance.

Endurance athletes and endurance events seem larger than life. Certainly, endurance sport is a more grandiose topic than any book can ever hope to cover completely. I've taken a stab at covering the topic broadly, although I know that every endurance athlete has a unique perspective on the sports that he or she practices. I can only represent the range of those perspectives, not every point of view. I hope reading this book will help you understand your experience of endurance sport.

THE EVENTS

PART

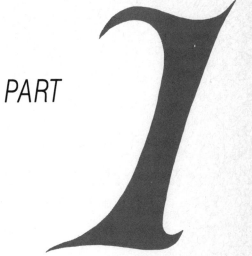

THE RUGGED INDIVIDUAL EVENTS

*I*T IS August 3, 1974, and the Tevis Cup Ride, a 100-mile horse race across the rugged Sierra Nevadas, is in full swing. Picture a bearded man with shoulder-length, sun-bleached blond hair calmly standing in line at a mandatory stopping point in the endurance ride to have his vital signs checked by a veterinarian. The flaxen-haired gent, Gordy Ainsleigh, was not pausing to have his steed examined, mind you, but standing in line to be checked himself. Rather than ride a horse, as did all the other competitors, he was pitting himself against the horses and the mountainous terrain in this 100-mile trail ride, and the officials probably figured the human runner was no less worthy of humane treatment than were the equine entrants. It is in such incongruous, humble circumstances that the Western States 100-Mile Endurance Run was born.* Today a finisher's belt buckle from the Western States 100-Miler, a humans-only footrace, is one of the most coveted trophies in endurance athletics. So many athletes wish to achieve the formidable feat of running 100 miles across a mountain range that safety and environmental concerns require limitation of the field by qualifications and a lottery.

Other 100-mile trail runs have sprung up, each with its own unique character. For instance, the Wasatch 100-Miler, in Utah, features climbs so steep that much of the race has to be done on hands and knees. To call the mountain views of California's Pacific Crest Trail 100-Miler awesome would be an understatement. Another 100-mile race traverses Death Valley.

The Western States 100-Miler is merely one of many endurance events that pits human abilities against the very grandeur of our planet. And not all the rugged individual events are footraces either.

Marathons, ultramarathons, long-distance swims, assaults on moun-

---

*In 1985 the Western States course was lengthened a few miles because an accurate survey revealed it had been short.

tain peaks—these are the endurance events that humans do under their own power. No animal or machine carries the athlete along—he or she competes alone against terrain, gravity, the clock, and other people. Here we have endurance in its purest and most elemental form: contests of humans against the elements. The swim across the English Channel. The climb up Mount Everest. The Western States 100-Mile footrace.

Why do these events so capture our imagination? Perhaps it is because such challenges to the planet's unyielding forces are very near the edge of what is humanly possible. The contestants walk a fine line between insane foolhardiness and courageous, awe-inspiring strength. Endurance athletes have persevered until they have dropped from exhaustion. In 1984 Gabrielle Anderson-Scheiss, a Swiss contestant in the first woman's Olympic marathon, stumbled and barely finished before collapsing of heat exhaustion from the heat and humidity of Los Angeles.

Bodies have surrendered before minds were ready to throw in the towel. In a few cases endurance athletes have lost their lives in pursuit of the ultimate boundaries of human performance.

ULTRADISTANCE RUNNING

The Tarahumara Indians of Mexico are a tribe of runners. Although the games of present-day Tarahumaras suggest that their pre-Columbian ancestors may have engaged in competition, throughout the world, ultradistance running probably served largely spiritual or utilitarian purposes until relatively recent years. Long-distance running, as a sport, probably did not emerge much before the last 150 years or so.

Although the marathon was a major feature of the very first modern Olympics, in 1896, there is little evidence that ancient Olympians ever competed in running events at distances beyond a mile. Baron Pierre de Coubertin and others responsible for the birth of the modern Olympics were neoclassicists. As did many of their nineteenth-century contemporaries involved in the fields of music, art, architecture, and literature, the founders of the Olympics looked to the ancient Greeks and Romans for their inspiration and often for their ideas. In the case of the marathon, Olympic founders either failed to plagiarize accurately or allowed themselves some poetic license. Despite the fact that the marathon has become the final event and crowning glory of the modern Olympics, it must be remembered that the 26.2-mile footrace commemorates a run by Pheidippides, a courier, not an athlete. That legendary Greek was doing his job—perhaps performing his sacred duty—when he allegedly ran himself to death in order to convey the message to Athens that the Persians had been defeated at the plains of Marathon. A courageous feat of endurance, but not sport.

Doubtless many readers of this book have run marathons and lived to tell the tale. A marathon is formidable, but not necessarily fatal. Scholars of ancient Greece are uncertain whether Pheidippides or some other courier did the run, and whether the messenger died as a result of the run. Indeed, the only reason the run was even difficult for him may have been that he had completed a 150-mile run just a day before.

In the last decade or so, millions of runners have completed a marathon, and only a handful, people with heart conditions, died. The explanation for this obviously lies in systematic training and other preparation for an athletic event.

Properly trained, humans are excellent distance runners. Many other species are faster in a sprint, but over the long haul humans very often triumph. As psychiatrist and running therapist Thaddeus Kostrubala has pointed out, one of the reasons the human species has survived is that entire hunting bands of our primordial ancestors could run for hours, even days, chasing prey that could easily beat us in a short race. When the elk or bison dropped from exhaustion, the humans still had something left and moved in for the kill.

As suited as we are to distance running, few people actually do it to the extreme, and we still marvel at the achievements of ultradistance runners. What are the ultimate challenges to runners? Regardless of the distance, for many runners the carrot of a personal record, or PR, can motivate performance. A small number of elite athletes can still advance our species' collective ability by pushing world records lower and lower. Even without speed barriers to break, merely moving long distances across the earth's surface is an impressive challenge in its own right. Ultradistance races take on a mystique and status larger than the athletes who do them. There is a fascination with brute distance. That is why in the six-day race endurance and distance tell the whole story.

The first heyday of six-day racing occurred between 1870 and 1900, when Irish, English, and American athletes popularly known as "pedestrians" chased each other around oval indoor tracks, while the fans vented nationalistic fervor or plotted foul play in order to win wagers. Edward Payson Weston, the first of the great American pedestrians, earlier had distinguished himself by such feats as walking 443 miles from Boston to Washington, D.C., to attend Lincoln's first inauguration. In 1867, after Civil War service as a Union spy, Weston won a $10,000 bet by traversing the 1,326 miles from Portland, Maine, to

Chicago in twenty-six days. In 1874, Weston became the first athlete to break the 500-mile mark in six days. It took the entire police force of Newark and the New Jersey state militia to protect Weston from New York thugs hired by gamblers to sabotage his effort, but Weston attained the 500-mile mark with approximately 25 minutes of his 144 hours remaining. (Weston continued his athletic career until the age of seventy-four, when in 1913 he walked the 1,500 miles between New York City and Minneapolis, Minnesota. He died at age ninety, on May 13, 1929.)

Back when Chester A. Arthur was president, a dollar was made of honest-to-God silver and was worth 100 cents. In fact, in those days, the U.S. Treasury would redeem folding money in gold. Thus, the $20,000 prizes offered six-day racers—who in the 1880s competed at such prestigious venues as Madison Square Garden—might be comparable to a $500,000 race purse today. In those days, before baseball and football had become big-time, the six-day footrace was major sport.

With a $19,000 carrot in front of him, George Haezel of England went 220 yards past the 600-mile barrier in a six-day effort of 1882. Philadelphian James Albert advanced the record to 621 miles in 1888. Later that same year, George Littlewood of England set a six-day record of 623.75 miles. One of the most durable athletic records of modern history, Littlewood's mark stood until July 8, 1984—nearly a century later. (The record was so durable that its authenticity has been debated, despite the presence of thousands of critical witnesses, many of whom had bet money on the outcome.)

By 1888, interest—as well as gate receipts and prize money—for six-day racing had already begun a pitiful decline. By 1910, the six-day footrace was just a memory. As recently as April 1980, Tom Ostler lamented in *Runner's World*, "Six-day racing is a sport now as defunct as ice baseball and horseback boxing." A few months later, however, the six-day footrace rose from the dead. In July 1980, ultradistance runner Don Choi staged the first modern six-day race in Woodside, California. Today the sport of six-day running is very much alive and well on Randall's Island, New York, among other places. Even the "Astley belt," an award that was previously offered to six-day racers by England's Lord Astley, has been revived. The new Astley Belt Six-Day Race of 1985 was staged in El Cajon, California. Stu Mittleman, a graduate student at New York's Columbia University, won that California race with a distance of 534 miles.

The modern six-day race has an international character. Races have been held in Nottingham, England; La Rochelle, France; San Diego; New York; and Colac, Australia. The contestants come from all over the world. The 1983 New York Road Runners Six-Day Race on Randall's Island was won by a New Zealander, Siegfried Bauer, and the thirty-one contestants in New York's 1984 race included runners of seven different nationalities. A Greek stadium attendant, twenty-eight-year-old Yiannis Kouros, won the New York six-day race in 1984, setting the new world record of 635 miles and 1,023 yards.

Most six-day runners use a slow-but-steady, grind-it-out strategy; but not Kouros. Remarkably, along the way Kouros ran a 2:52 marathon for the first 26.2 miles, established new world records for forty-eight hours (266 miles) and seventy-two hours (359.76 miles), despite blistering heat, oppressive humidity, and thunderstorms.

At the same six-day race, a thirty-six-year-old housewife from England, Eleanor Adams, set a new women's record of 426 miles, 278 yards. In marked contrast to the pedestrian heyday of the 1880s, Eleanor Adams received no prize and Yiannis Kouros received only $2,500 for winning and an extra $5,000 for the world record.

Still, the six-day race has entered the twentieth century. Though most of the six-day racers still know one another, in the manner of marathoners before the 1960s, clearly the sport is growing. The extreme physical demands of this sport will probably always limit participation, but the recognition for the athletes may come as a consequence of new performance records.

Other old events may be revived, too. In 1928 and 1929 C. C. Pyle, an athletic promoter extraordinaire, organized transcontinental footraces, popularly known as "Corn and Bunion Derbies." The 1929 race included stages from 25 to 72 miles in length, during a period of just eighty days. The April 1, 1929, *New York Times* estimated that half a million spectators lined the route as Ed Gardner, of Seattle, Washington, won the first 25.1-mile stage from New York's Columbus Circle to Newark. Gardner's margin of victory for that stage was just 25 yards. He averaged a 4:45 pace, if Pyle's measurement of the distance is to be believed. Gardner was not among the 3,635-mile race's nineteen finishers, though. Johnny Salo beat his nearest competitor by less than three minutes to win the race with a cumulative time of 525:57.20.

In the 1929 race, the first fifteen finishers shared $60,000 of prize money with $25,000 going to the first finisher. (At June 1984 prices the total purse would be worth over $363,000.) Several modern promoters have tried to resurrect Pyle's event, and perhaps somebody will succeed. There now is a community of ultradistance runners willing and able to take up that challenge again.

Although the prize money of ultradistance running's salad days has not yet returned, the talent has been reborn. Shortly after the record-breaking 1984 New York Road Runners Six-Day, Fred Lebow ebulliently predicted that the new men's record, which took ninety-six years to arrive, would stand for another hundred years. He also predicted that the women's mark would soon break the 500-mile barrier. Score one point for Lebow and one point against him. He underestimated the skills of Yiannis Kouros and was right on target with his projections for womankind. Demonstrating noteworthy abilities to recover, Yiannis Kouros broke his own record within the year at a six-day race in Colac, Australia. At the same race, Eleanor Adams ran 501 miles, 129 yards, increasing her own world record by almost 75 miles.

Kouros exceeded his previous world record by only 362 yards, but clearly this clone of the legendary Pheidippides could have done even better. With more than an hour remaining in the race, Kouros stopped just short of his New York record, because he believed that the race promoter had broken some promises. The main grievances were the condition of the track and financial arrangements. Kouros alleged that he had been shortchanged on promised appearance money and an automobile, which initially had been offered as an incentive to set the record. He resumed running only when urged to do so by relatives and other members of the local Greek community. In the best traditions of the feisty nineteenth-century six-day runners, he was feuding with management over money and limiting productivity accordingly.

In an article that appeared in the January 1985 issue of *Ultrarunning* magazine, Dan Brannen speculated that Yiannis Kouros "is the only runner for whom an accusation of cheating eventually became an honor." Although Kouros is a 2:24 marathoner, race officials could not believe that he ran the entire 145 miles, when he outpaced all competitors by three hours in the 1984 Spartathlon. His subsequent performance in the next year's Spartathlon and in other races was meticulously monitored, and it was so superior to ordinary ultradistance running that the skeptics are now believers. Most of them concede that he ran every mountainous inch of the Spartathlon's Sparta-to-Athens course.

Critics of the six-day race call it a sport for masochists, cultists, and eccentrics. And often the scene at the six-day race does have a rather bizarre quality. For instance, Nathan Whiting, a poet who sports baggy shorts and a scraggly beard reminiscent of the fried noodles at a Chinese restaurant, often carries a parasol while running. At the 1984 race at Randall's Island, some contestants tried to "concentrate" their sleep by taking catnaps in a small white, egg-shaped isolation chamber cum waterbed, made by the Ova Corporation. Trishful Cherns enlivened the 1984 New York race by briefly running with an orange traffic cone on his head.

Despite the sometimes amusing conduct and strange costumes—e.g., pajamas, floppy hats, baggy pants, pockets filled with ice cubes—the sport of six-day running is serious. True, it isn't normal to see someone eat a bowl of soup while encircling a track, but the contestants are living for six days on that track, not just running. They have to eat and drink somewhere, even though they manage to do precious little sleeping. Carrying a parasol makes more sense than not carrying one, if you anticipate running for days in the blazing sun. So what if Yiannis Kouros runs in broken-down shoes with the toe boxes cut out; naked toes are less likely to suffer the perennial runner's curse, black toenail. And as Kouros explains, "There are memories in these shoes."

Still, some short-distance runners are concerned that such antics will damage the yuppie image of the sport of running. To many runners the six-day race seems a freak show. Perhaps most irritating to these critics are the vivid descriptions of hallucinations given by six-day runners, but allowances should be made for that too. The six-day runners are experiencing perceptions that most people never will; of course they want to describe them.

In any case, the idiosyncrasies of the contestants will likely encourage rather than deter media coverage. ABC's "Nightline" reported live on the 1983 New York six-day, including commentary while running by contestant Stu Mittleman. *The New York Times* and magazines such as *Ultrasport* and *Ultrarunning* also report on six-day racing. Media coverage will encourage the growth of ultradistance running, albeit more modestly than it did the growth of the marathon. Already six-day racing has an international sanctioning body, and a race calendar is slowly evolving for the small community of ultradistance runners who pursue this extremely demanding sport.

The six-day runners might be on the lunatic fringe, but they may be running for all of us. Most humans will never attempt a race of 144 hours' duration, but Yiannis Kouros carried the torch of human endurance just a few miles farther when he set his records.

EVEREST

Farther than anybody else is one thing, but how about higher? Although it takes an expedition—a first-rate team—to conquer Everest, the sixty or so men and women who have stood on the top of the world walked there under their own power. There is no question that Himalayan climbing requires individual endurance and courage. Everest has claimed the lives of approximately fifty climbers. Certainly each death was an individual sacrifice to the relentless drive to push back the boundaries of our collective endurance.

Why the fascination with Everest? Everest is a giant among mountains; it is higher than any other mountain on earth. Standing 29,028 feet above sea level, Everest, or Chomolungma, as the Tibetans call it, is a behemoth of a mountain.*

A second reason for the fascination with Everest is its inaccessibility. Until 1855, the world at large did not even know Everest existed. The Sherpa inhabitants of the Himalayan region could see Everest, but they had no idea of its preeminence among the world's mountains. From their vantage point below, Everest appeared smaller than other nearby peaks. The height of Everest could not be determined without surveying instruments, and with crude nineteenth-century measurements the stature of Everest was incorrectly calculated as 29,002 feet. We now know that Everest is 26 feet taller than the first measurements indicated.†

After the Western world finally learned of Everest and its stature, various groups and individuals wished to explore that area or attempt to climb the mountain, but the Nepalese and Tibetan governments prevented foreign expeditions from entering the region.

Relying on disguises and subterfuge, Indian army captain J. B. L. Noel illegally explored the vicinity of Everest in 1913. It was not until 1921 that Tibet authorized an expedition to survey Everest. Two English organizations, the Royal Geographic Society and the Alpine Club, sponsored the expedition.

The renowned British mountaineer George L. Mallory, a member of the 1921 expedition, gave a third reason that the world is so fascinated with Everest. In his book *Men Against Everest* Mallory warned, "We must remember that the highest of mountains is capable of severity, a severity so awful and so fatal that the wiser sort of men do well to think and tremble even on the threshold of their high endeavor."

Mallory's words were morbidly prophetic. In a 1922 expedition, he survived an avalanche on Everest that took the lives of seven Sherpa porters. Then, in an assault on Everest's summit during a 1924 expedition, both Mallory and his climbing partner, Andrew Irvine, an

---

*The Nepalese (who live to the south of the mountain) call Everest *Sagarmatha,* "Goddess Mother of the world." The name Everest commemorates the work of Sir George Everest, the predecessor of British Surveyor General Andrew Waugh, whose 1855 expedition determined that the mountain was a separate peak and the highest in the world. The practice of the Geodetic Survey of India, over which Waugh presided, was to use the local name for mountains. When it was first surveyed, however, no local name was known for the mountain.

†Interestingly, Everest is actually growing, at the rate of about 36 feet per century. Rocks brought back from the top indicate conclusively that the mountain has been thrusting up from the ocean floor during the past 20 million years. The top of Everest was once under water!

Oxford student, perished somewhere above 28,000 feet. Indeed, the hapless pair, who disappeared into a mist that shrouded the higher reaches of Everest, may have made it to the top. We have no way of knowing.

Conditions on this mountain are harsh to the extreme. Professor N. E. Odell, who searched in vain for Mallory and Irvine, describes the upper part of Everest as "the remotest and least hospitable spot on earth." Blizzards, subzero temperatures, and howling winds can blow a climber off the mountain. Everest expeditions must end before the monsoon season brings its annual deluge of snow. On a sunny day the glare can easily cause snow blindness. Hidden, yawning crevasses can instantly swallow the climber who missteps. Many climbers have been buried alive in one of the frequent avalanches that characterize the constantly shifting Khombu Icefall of Everest. And, as if these problems were not enough, the altitude is so great that for almost all climbers the air is too thin to support exertion without the aid of heavy tanks of oxygen.

During the years from 1924 until World War II, five climbing parties attempted to reach the summit of Everest. All of these failed, one fatally. Maurice Wilson, an English devotee of yoga, believed that fasting to summon his internal spiritual strength would enable him to succeed on a solo climb of Everest in 1934. One year later, Eric Shipton's expedition found the novice mountaineer's body inside the tattered shreds of his tent. Wilson's desire to perform could not compensate for inexperience and lack of training, and that seems to be generally true of hazardous endurance challenges.

During World War II no resources were available for Everest assaults. Then in 1947, Earl Denman, a Canadian, with somewhat better climbing background than Wilson, failed at about 23,000 feet in an unauthorized attempt. Poorly equipped, Denman was defeated by the harsh weather, despite a gutsy solo attempt. Nonetheless, he climbed with an immortal. Denman was accompanied partway by a Sherpa named Tenzing Norgay, who was to feature prominently in numerous other expeditions and ultimately would share the first conquest of Everest with Sir Edmund Hillary.

Between 1950 and 1952 there were seven Everest attempts, including an American, two British, two Swiss, and a Russian expedition, and a solo climb by a Dane, R. Becker-Larsen. In all, nine brave mountaineers died on these missions, and nobody stood on top of the world.

Post–World War II Everest ambitions were hampered to some extent by the revolution in China. The Communist Chinese troops occupying Tibet would not allow climbers to approach the mountain from the north. Although Nepal had adopted a more permissive policy, the conventional wisdom about Everest had always been that the mountain's defenses could not be breached from the south.

Then, in 1952, Eric Shipton's fifth British expedition, which included New Zealander Edmund Hillary, made some discoveries about the mountain's southern defenses. On the basis of their exploration, the Shipton team proposed that there was a climbable route from Nepal. This possible route would proceed up a deep ravine known as the Western Cwm, and continue onto the face of an adjacent mountain called Lhotse. Weather permitting, the climbers then would climb up over a rib of rock (the Geneva Spur) to a dip called the South Col. From the South Col, the path would be up to the South Summit, which from below would falsely appear to be the top, and then up an apparently treacherous ridge (above 28,000 feet) to the top. Unfortunately, three days of heavy snowfall prevented Shipton's expedition from testing its theory.

Finally, in 1953, a massive expedition led by a senior British army officer, Lord John Hunt, was dispatched to Everest by the Himalayan Committee. At age forty-two, Hunt was a superb mountain climber with a distinguished war record that included a stint as top mountaineering trainer of Britain's commando force. His background as a military leader may well have been ideal for his role on Everest, because he commanded a small army of 350 porters, 20 Sherpas, and 10 principal climbers, including Hillary and Norgay.

As had the 1952 Swiss expedition, the Hunt group would follow the southern route first suggested by Shipton. The crux of Hunt's strategy for his Everest campaign was to get sufficient oxygen, food, mountaineering equipment, and climbers high enough on Everest to permit as many as three assaults on the top by two pairs of acclimatized mountaineers. It was critical that the summit pairs be supported well enough so that at about 28,000 feet they could begin their thrusts adequately equipped and in a rested and fit condition. Accordingly, Hunt's Everest crusade set out from Katmandu on March 10, 1953, with over seven tons of baggage. After a trek of approximately 125 miles, a base camp was established at Thyangboche. From base camp, the climbers experimented with and trained themselves in the use of the oxygen by climbing nearby peaks at about 20,000 feet. Finally, using a leapfrog procedure, the principal climbers opened paths to successively higher camps, and then descended to lead teams of Sherpas carrying heavy loads ever upward.

The equipment relays were dangerous and difficult, particularly across the avalanche-prone Khombu Icefall. The climbers and Sherpas carried heavy ladders up the mountain to use as bridges across unavoidable crevasses. In all, the Sherpa caravans carried 750 pounds of cargo up 26,000 feet to the South Col, the jumping-off point for the summit assaults.

After weeks of building ever higher camps, on May 24, 1953, one of the summit pairs, Charles Evans and Tom Bordillon, were ready to leave the South Col (Camp VII) for the summit. Mechanical problems with their oxygen apparatus caused Evans and Bordillon to make a late departure. Their support crew, which consisted of Colonel Hunt and the Sherpa Da Namgyal, had left earlier and reached 27,350 feet. At that altitude Hunt and Da Namgyal left oxygen bottles to be used by the second assault pair, Hillary and Norgay. Climbing strongly after their frustrating mechanical delay, Evans and Bordillon caught up with Hunt and Da Namgyal, who, having accomplished their support mission, headed for lower altitudes. Evans and Bordillon attained the South Summit (28,720 feet high) but could not climb the remaining 500 feet. They had arrived too late in the day and too short of oxygen to reach the peak and return safely. Evans and Bordillon were forced to retreat, to rest up for another attempt if the second assault team failed too.

On May 28, 1953, Norgay and Hillary climbed from the South Col to 27,900 feet, supported by George Lowe, Alfred Gregory, and the Sherpa Ang Nyima. From that height, the support personnel returned to lower altitudes. Meanwhile, Hillary and Norgay established a high-altitude camp and rested from 2:30 P.M. until the next morning. They arose at 4:00 A.M. on the twenty-ninth and melted snow on a Primus stove; this was absolutely critical to obtain fluids to prevent dehydration, a persistent problem for climbers using oxygen at high altitudes. Hillary was forced to use the flame to thaw out his boots, which had frozen. They checked their oxygen sets and departed for the peak at 6:30 A.M. Cutting steps in the glacier on their way up, the team reached the South Summit at 9:00 A.M.

Weather conditions were ideal. Norgay and Hillary began their ascent of the final ridge. They knew that they had to avoid putting any weight on the cornices of snow overhanging the right side of the ridge. Those shelves of snow could give way and drop them 10,000 feet down the side of the Kangshung Face. But Norgay and Hillary did not know whether they could move efficiently on the well-supported snow on the left side of the ridge. If the snow was soft, the going would be tough and the length of exertion required would have made the climb impossible in the oxygen-deprived environment. Their oxygen tanks would be depleted before they could reach the top and return. No human had ever stepped on that ridge before—and lived to talk about it. They had no way to know in advance.

Fortunately, the snow was firmly crystallized. They were able to belay each other up the ridge comfortably and carefully, until they reached a 40-foot-high rock step.* Although Hillary tells us this obstacle was "smooth and holdless," at a lower altitude it would have provided no more than an interesting challenge to a thoroughly rested, expert rock-climber. However, as Hillary put it in Sir John Hunt's 1954 book *The Conquest of Everest*, "At this altitude it [the rock] might spell the difference between success and failure . . . here it was a barrier beyond our feeble strength to overcome."

Rather than attempt to climb directly up the rock, Hillary wedged himself into a crack between the rock and an overhanging snow cornice. With his back to the rock, Hillary dug the front spikes of his crampons into the ice of the cornice. In his chapter of Hunt's book, Hillary described this awkward, exhausting maneuver:

> Taking advantage of every little rock hold and all the force of knee, shoulder and arms I could muster, I literally cramponed backwards up the crack, with a fervent prayer that the cornice would remain attached to the rock. Despite the considerable effort involved, my progress, although slow, was steady, and as Tenzing paid out the rope I inched my way upward until I could finally reach over the top of the rock and drag myself out of the crack onto a wide ledge. For a few moments I lay regaining my breath and for the first time really felt the fierce determination that nothing now could stop our reaching the top. I took a firm stance on the ledge and signaled to Tenzing to come on up. As I heaved hard on the rope Tenzing wriggled his way up the crack and finally collapsed exhausted at the top like a giant fish when it has just been hauled from the sea after a terrible struggle.

Then the pair resumed their seemingly endless trudge up this final ridge, chipping steps in the snow as they went. Just as their physical resources had dwindled to almost nothing, Hillary noticed that the never-ending upward ridge was beginning to drop away. To conquer Everest, it remained only to climb up a short, slender ridge of snow. In Hillary's own words, "A few more whacks of the ice ax in the firm snow and we stood on top."

Years later Hillary wrote in the preface to Major H. P. S. Ahluwalia's book *The Faces of Everest*, "Tenzing and I stepped on the summit of Everest on May 29, 1953. I felt no great surge of joy and exaltation—only a mixture of more subdued feelings. There was a quiet satisfaction that we had finally made it; a tinge of surprise that I, Ed Hillary, should be standing here on top when so many good men

---

*To *belay* is to protect a climber's movements with a safety rope anchored to an object or another climber.

had failed. Behind it all my brain constantly churned out its familiar arithmetic—how many litres of oxygen did we have left? Could we get down safely?"

Using their remaining oxygen—plus the bottles left by Hunt's support team at 23,500 feet—Tenzing and Hillary were just able to complete their descent to the South Col as they ran out of the life-giving gas. There they were reunited with climbers George Lowe and Wilfrid Noyce.

The main body of the expedition, on the slopes below, had to wait for the return of the summit climbers before they learned of the victory. If the summit assault succeeded, Noyce was supposed to signal that news to the mountaineers below by placing sleeping bags on the snow in a T shape. However, sunset prevented reception of that visual message. When the victors finally arrived with the fabulous news, James Morris, a correspondent for the London *Times* who had accompanied the expedition, climbed down from advance base to base camp to file his story by wireless. His perfectly timed dispatch reached England at just the moment to become a dramatic focal point of the celebration of Queen Elizabeth's coronation.

The Hunt expedition had been widely publicized and followed anxiously throughout the world. News that Everest had been conquered was electrifying. We finally had become masters of this planet.

While on the summit of Everest, Hillary viewed Makalu, a nearby unclimbed peak. He reports that "even on top of Everest the mountaineering instinct was sufficiently strong to cause me to spend some moments conjecturing as to whether a route up that mountain might not exist." One might conclude that Hillary was a glutton for punishment, but his reaction also strikes close to the very heart of endurance. Many endurance athletes, at their moment of supreme triumph, begin to ponder the next challenge.

Taking this beyond the single athlete, we see the conquest of Everest as merely an inspiration to others to take up new endurance challenges. In 1954, just one year after the first conquest of Everest, Lord Hunt wrote, "The ascent of Everest seems to have stirred the spirit of adventure latent in every human breast . . . someday Everest will be climbed again." Indeed the mountain has been reclimbed. Swiss, American, Indian, Japanese, Italian, Chinese, Austrian, German, and other British climbers have all stood on the peak. In 1970, a Japanese ski champion, Y. Miura, accompanied by a camera crew, climbed to the South Col and descended using skis and a parachute. On May 16, 1975, Japanese climber Junko Tabei became the first woman to conquer Everest. In spring 1975, an expedition from the People's Republic of China put nine climbers on the summit, conducted much useful scientific research up there, and made the mountain just a bit taller by planting a 3-meter survey pole.

Hunt less optimistically also wrote, "It [an assault on Everest] may well be attempted without oxygen, although I do not rate the chances of success very high at present." In this instance Hunt clearly underestimated human endurance. Shortly after noon, May 8, 1978, Reinhold Messner and Peter Habeler of Austria were on Everest, climbing at 28,600 feet, without oxygen tanks. Messner writes of the experience, "Breathing became such a strenuous business that we scarcely have strength left to go on. Every ten or fifteen steps we collapse into the snow to rest, then crawl on again. My mind seems almost to have ceased to function. I simply go on climbing automatically."

Messner and Habeler climbed on until they reached the summit, realizing Messner's dream to conquer Everest "by fair means," that is, without carrying oxygen. Climbing from base camp to the summit, they never once resorted to oxygen equipment. The pair returned safely, with no immediately apparent physiological damage. Another challenge had succumbed to the unstoppable drive of human endurance.

THE ENGLISH CHANNEL

It was neither fighting in the hedgerows nor on the beaches that kept Napoleon and Hitler from invading Great Britain; it was a natural moat, the English Channel. That is why a simple accomplishment, successfully swimming the English Channel, can utterly rivet our attention. At the English Channel's narrowest point, a mere 21 miles of water separate Dover, England, from its nearest French neighbor, Cap Gris Nez. But it is turbulent water, with tricky tides and currents. Cold, too; very rarely much over 60 degrees Fahrenheit, usually much colder. Suitable perhaps for porpoises or walruses, with their layers of insulating fat, but almost guaranteed to cause fatal hypothermia to most human swimmers. "Only" 21 miles, a short stretch compared to other distances over water, but it might as well be a thousand miles.

Until August 1875, nobody had swum across the Channel, although a few had tried and some had managed to swim partway or get across doing something similar to swimming. It is alleged that a French prisoner of war, Jean-Marie Salett, escaped from a British prison ship anchored off Dover by swimming to Boulogne in the summer of 1815. It seems unlikely, however, that he could have swum the entire distance without food and drinking water. Another Frenchman, a veteran of Napoleon's army, actually crossed the Channel before 1875; but he cheated by frequently taking ten-minute rests in his guide boat. On December 20, 1862, an English sailor named Hoskins successfully doggie-paddled across the Channel on a bundle of straw. Amid much fanfare, including a sendoff by a twenty-piece band, J. B. Johnson, a flamboyant English swimmer, set out across the Channel in 1873. Johnson's attempt lasted about an hour, at which time the shivering, would-be champion clambered aboard his guide boat.

During the spring of 1875, an American inventor, Captain Paul Boynton, made two attempts to cross the Channel wearing his invention, a rubber lifesaving suit that had built-in flotation. He wished to test and publicize his contraption. On his second attempt, on May 28, 1875, Boynton successfully crossed the Channel from Cap Gris Nez to Foreland, England.

Although it is well documented that Hoskins and Boynton actually did cross the Channel, both men relied on some form of flotation device to do so. It remained for Captain Matthew Webb, a master of sailing vessels, to become the first person to swim across the Channel legitimately, without the assistance of a boat or a buoyant device.

Born in Shropshire, England, Webb had taught himself to swim at the age of nine. His attitude toward swimming appeared to have been fearless, if not downright foolhardy. The Royal Humane Society decorated Webb for bravery when, as a sailor aboard a Cunard mail packet, the *Russia*, he jumped into 45-degree water to attempt a rescue of a shipmate who had fallen overboard. The *Russia* was steaming at over 14 knots at the time, and it took more than an hour for the ship to turn and retrieve him. Most humans who spend that length of time in cold water die, and Webb was lucky even to be spotted in the rough water at all. Although the brave Webb dove repeatedly in attempts to locate his shipmate, the other sailor was lost at sea. Eventually Webb's disregard for the dangers of the water would cost him his life, too, but not before he had conquered the English Channel.

If ever a swimmer was suited to tame the English Channel, it was Matthew Webb. Another Englishman, J. B. Johnson, who had failed to cross the Channel in 1873, was a "bathhouse" swimmer; that is, he did his swimming in the confines of a warm, calm swimming pool. Johnson may have been capable of swimming the distance required in a pool, but workouts at the bathhouse left him unprepared for the tides, currents, and cold, choppy waters of the English Channel. Matthew Webb, on the other hand, was a rough-water swimmer. He knew that he could succeed where Johnson had failed, in open waters, so Webb set the Channel as his mark.

The young seafarer took a bold step to accomplish his goal. He set about raising the money it would cost to obtain such logistic support as a guide boat and handlers. First he wagered ten pounds, at odds, that he could swim the 18 miles of the Thames River, from Blackwall Pier to Gravesend. He won his bet easily. Assisted by the current, Webb accomplished that swim in a mere five hours—not a bad swim, considering that the crawl had not yet been invented and Webb used the breaststroke.

Webb did more than just win a bet when he swam down the Thames; he also obtained a sponsor. Frank Buckland, publisher of *Land and Water* magazine, met Webb and recognized the publicity value of his proposed Channel swim. By publicizing the attempt, Buckland convinced members of the London business community to pledge several hundred pounds, which would be paid to Webb if he successfully crossed the Channel.

At 5:00 P.M. on August 12, 1875, Webb set out for France. Unfortunately, the seas at the hour of departure were decidedly against Webb; his relatively slow breaststroke was not powerful enough to prevent the current from sweeping him up the Channel parallel to the English shore. After six hours and forty-nine minutes, approaching foul weather forced Webb and his support crew to abort their mission. Although Webb was still fit and strong when weather intervened, he almost certainly would have failed anyway. Sad to say, during almost seven hours of effort, the current had pulled him 18 miles up the English coast, as he stroked only 5 miles toward France.

After twelve days of recuperation and one other frustrating delay due to weather, at 12:56 P.M., on August 24, 1875, Webb again entered the water from Admiralty Pier. For twenty-one hours and forty-five minutes he stroked a zigzag course across the channel. In all, Webb's course probably covered at least 35 miles, as the tides and currents again carried him off the most direct route. For the early part of the historic swim the seas were calm. The water temperature that day averaged about 60 degrees Fahrenheit, balmy by Channel standards.

A reporter from *Land and Water* periodically swam alongside Webb to break the monotony. Webb's feedings during the swim were mostly hot liquids, such as coffee and beef tea, but he also took brandy and cod liver oil. Late in the swim he stopped to chew on raw meat.

As any endurance athlete might predict, the last portion of Webb's swim was the most difficult. But the cause of the problem was more than just the swimmer's exhaustion; the tide turned against him. After fourteen hours of swimming, Webb was only 4 miles off Cap Gris Nez; but during the cold predawn hours, when he most needed encouragement, the tide would not permit a landing. Worse yet, at that critical point, the wind picked up and the seas became choppy. During the next seven hours the tide carried Webb some thirteen miles up the French coast to Calais, as he made torturously slow progress toward land. He persevered though, and at the Calais Pier Webb was able to stumble ashore into the waiting arms of cheering spectators.

Webb was one of the earliest sports heroes to achieve any degree of wealth. Initially, admiring fans showered him with $45,000 in gifts, including $25,000 from the Prince of Wales. Webb later earned as much as $2,000 for such endurance stunts as swimming in a tank for seventy-four hours, but his box-office appeal steadily waned. During his period of popularity, Webb married an English woman, with whom he had two children. When his earning powers declined in England, he transplanted his family to the United States, where his diminishing fame barely enabled him to earn a living. To reestablish his notoriety, he plotted a spectacular swim across the Niagara River in the angry rapids below the falls.

On an August day in 1883 the thirty-five-year-old conqueror of the English Channel dove into the turbulent Niagara River on the U.S. side. To the horror of the hundreds of spectators watching from the suspension bridge across the river, Webb was pulled under by the churning water within minutes of entry. In a manner of speaking, he did make it across the river. Four days after he disappeared, his body washed up on the Canadian shore, 5 miles downstream of his U.S. departure point. The very fearlessness that had made Webb a hero and a splendid endurance swimmer ultimately cost him his life.

Webb's pathetic demise in no way diminishes the magnitude or the importance of his earlier endurance achievement. Although many tried, nobody was able to duplicate Webb's Channel swim for the next thirty-six years. In 1911, Thomas Burgess succeeded, on his fourteenth attempt, to cross the Channel, in a time of 22:35, or just shy of an hour longer than Webb. Then more than a decade elapsed before the moat was crossed again. Between 1922 and 1926 several swimmers successfully crossed the Channel, including two who, in 1923, went in the reverse direction—from France to England. Now it is generally believed that swimming from France to England is easier than doing it the way Webb did, although Penny Dean, the current record holder, disagrees. In any event, the two swimmers who started from France crossed the Channel in record time. One of them, Argentine swimmer Enrico Tiraboschi, crossed in a time of 16:33. Only days later the other, American Charles Toth, crossed in 16:58.

Perhaps the most notable of all Channel swimmers was Gertrude Ederle, the daughter of a German immigrant who owned a small delicatessen in New York City. Gertrude Ederle was called "Trudy" by her friends and by the throng that showered her with tickertape upon her triumphant return to New York. There was ample reason to honor her. Not only was she the first woman to conquer the Channel, but she also set a new record in the process—14:31. (By 1926, when Ederle set her record, most Channel swimmers were using the crawl, an efficient, powerful stroke unknown in Webb's time.)

During the crossing, eighteen-year-old Trudy magnificently demonstrated her courage and assertiveness. Late in the endurance swim her handlers became alarmed by worsening sea conditions. They pleaded for her to quit. Without missing a stroke, Trudy replied, "What for?"

In 1927 the English Channel Swimming Association was formed to authenticate the claims of previous Channel swimmers and to sanction new swims. It provides official observers to ride the support boats and enforces the rules against such cheating as hanging on the boat. The association also maintains a list of qualified boat captains to act as guides.

Ernst Vierkotter's time of 12:40, set in August 1926, stood as the record until 1950. As is the case with so many athletic records, Vierkotter's mark fell victim to organized competition. In 1950 the *London Daily Mail* sponsored the first of a series of cross-Channel races that occurred each year of that decade except 1952. The first race in the series (1950) was won by an Egyptian army officer, Hassan Abd-el-Rheim, in the record time of 10:50. His victory presaged a decade of preeminence in endurance swimming for Egyptian athletes, who were sponsored and generously rewarded for their success by King Farouk. The 1950s, the golden age of Channel swimming, also saw the success of Greta Anderson, an American woman who beat all other men and women in the cross-Channel races of both 1957 and 1958.

Since the 1950s, several athletes have done the conventional Channel swimmer one better by completing double crossings. The first double crosser was Argentinian Antonio Abertondo, who in September 1961 swam from England to France and back in a total time of 43:10. Using a course and timetable plotted by computer to optimize changes of tide, Ted Erikson, an American chemist, made three double-crossing attempts in 1965. Cold water had halted an earlier try in 1964. His first two attempts of 1965 failed also. But the third try that year was a charm. That time Erikson had perfect weather and allowed his experienced boat captain, Peter Winter, to alter the computer-designed course as necessary. Erikson's round trip set a record of 30:03 that since has been bettered twice by Canadian Cindy Nicholas. Her best time is an almost unbelievable 18:55, which she swam on August 28, 1982.

Ted Erikson's twenty-six-year-old son, Jon, became the first swimmer to complete a triple crossing of the Channel on August 11–12, 1981. Previously, at age fourteen, Jon Erikson had become the youngest male swimmer to cross the Channel, but that record has since been

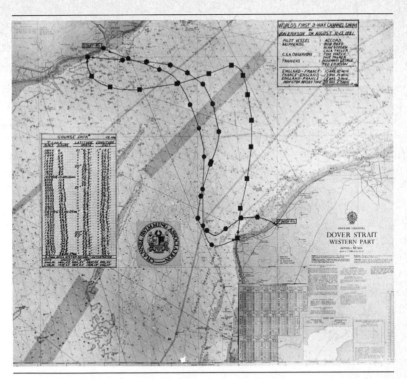

Nautical chart of the Channel triple crossing.

COURTESY OF TED ERIKSON

taken away by still younger swimmers. Like his father before him, Jon also briefly held the speed record for the fastest double crossing. The time for Jon's triple crossing was 38:27.

In a little over a century the phenomenal achievement of Captain Webb has been improved upon substantially. Impressive age records have been set. (Youngest Channel swimmer, Marcus Hooper of Eltham, England, age 12 years and 53 days; oldest swimmer, Ashby Harper of Albuquerque, New Mexico, 65 years and 332 days, time 13:52.) The record time for crossing the Channel was lowered to 7:40 by a twenty-three-year-old Californian, Penny Dean, on July 29, 1978. And, of course, the almost unbelievable double and triple crossings have already been mentioned.

Does all this mean that Webb's triumph was no big deal? Not at all. The nature of all endurance challenges is that they stretch human horizons. We have a tendency to become blasé when we read about records improving and performance barriers falling. Nonetheless, a marathon run in a time several minutes slower than the world record is still a remarkable feat. (Indeed, just finishing one is a pretty good trick.) The fact that Yiannis Kouros broke a ninety-six-year-old distance record in the six-day footrace doesn't mean that 623 miles (the old record) is no longer a great distance to run. When Messner and Habeler climbed Everest without oxygen, they didn't erase the triumph of Norgay and Hillary. Just because many swimmers have triumphed over the English Channel we can't assume that the next swim will be inconsequential. In fact, more than 1,100 swimmers have attempted a Channel crossing, but only about 20 percent have succeeded. The water stays just as cold, the opposite shore remains just as distant, and the physical effort of the next Channel swimmer will be just as great as Webb's. The only difference will be the knowledge that success is possible.

MAN AND BEAST

NOT ALL endurance athletes go it alone. Some people team up with four-legged partners to compete in unusual but increasingly popular contests.

The most familiar of these competitions are the endurance rides, long-distance horse races held over rugged terrain and ranging in distance from 25 to over 3,000 miles. An interesting twist on the horse race is the ride and tie, which pits teams of three—one horse, two people—against each other in a cross-country race. In colder climes, there are dog sled races long enough to tax driver and team to their limit.

Most unusual of all is the contest *between* human and beast—the occasional race between a human and a horse, which may be by turns amusing, surprising, and sad.

Sports that combine the efforts of humans and beasts frequently are well grounded in history. Often a competition will commemorate some colorful and dramatic historical event in which the endurance of both humans and animals saved the day. The ride and tie is such a race.

THE RIDE AND TIE

When rustlers made off with Captain William Emery's horses in the winter of 1873, Emery and his sixteen-year-old son, Charles, did what any self-respecting ranchers would do—they chased the varmints. The thieves had taken all but one horse from the Emery's Pine Valley, California, ranch. That presented father and son with a transportation problem. They both could have ridden the horse to the nearest stage-coach depot at La Mesa, but that would have been slow going, and they might easily have killed the poor beast over the 40-mile trek. Or they could have set out on foot, but walking is even slower than two on a horse, and after a few miles a man isn't much good for dealing with horse thieves. Instead, the Emerys used the ride-and-tie (or hitch-and-hike) method.

The name suggests the mode of travel. One human sets out on foot, the other on horseback. The rider travels ahead some distance, hitches up the horse, and proceeds on foot. Meanwhile, the other person walks or runs to the hitching spot, mounts up, and rides past the partner to the next agreed-upon hitching place. This tradeoff arrangement continues until all three have reached the destination. The horse—the only member of the team that has to cover the entire distance on foot—has plenty of time to rest and graze while waiting for the hiker, and the humans get transportation at least part of the way. It is an effective way of getting about when there are fewer horses than people, as in the case of the Emerys. They were able to reach the stagecoach station 40 miles from their ranch. From there, they rode the coach down to Mexico, where the rustlers were captured and promptly hanged.

The ride-and-tie method was apparently an established means of travel when Henry Fielding mentioned it in his 1743 novel, *Joseph Andrews*, but it was not until 1970 that the sport of ride and tie was born. Bud Johns, then director of public relations at Levi Strauss and Company, was set the task of founding a sporting event suitable for the blue-jeans manufacturer to sponsor. Johns recalled reading about the Emerys' ordeal at a Western history library and the thought struck him that a ride-and-tie race would fit the Levi's image better than any bowling tournament or tennis match.

By June 1971, Johns had produced the first Levi's Ride and Tie in St. Helena, California, drawing sixty-six teams in competition over a 25-mile course. The combination of endurance riding, distance running, race strategy, and team effort made for instant success, and ride and ties have sprung up at a phenomenal rate since then. There are more than 350 such events per year now, and the ride and tie has gone international. There are now competitions in both England and Germany.

At the first Levi's Ride and Tie, all the participants were novices. Nobody had staged a ride and tie before, so the event could hardly draw from a cadre of veteran contestants. Many entrants in the first race had disproportionately more experience in one of the two sports included in the event. For instance, Jim Larimer came to the first race as an endurance rider who had done very little running.

At thirty-eight, Larimer, who now earns his living as a manager for a savings and loan, has completed more than thirty-five endurance horse races. He rode in his first 100-mile race back in 1968, when he was twenty. Then in the spring of 1971 he and sixteen-year-old Hal Hall saw a poster for an unusual event called the Levi's Ride and Tie.

Hall and Larimer were attracted to the new 40-mile event, though neither of them was capable of running more than a mile. That first year, their training consisted of running around the streets of Auburn, California, where they lived. They were young, and they developed an intelligent strategy, so the disaster that one might have predicted did not occur. Their strategy was to walk the uphills and run the downhills, trying to make up time when they were on horseback.

Bill Posedel, an accomplished marathon runner from San Francisco, was also in the race. Posedel and his partner, John Holden, were both firemen in San Francisco. Larimer recollects: "I was pretty amazed that Posedel could run the hills." In spite of the fact that the two humans were novice runners, the team of Larimer, Hall, and a thoroughbred named Tabby did well. In fact, they did really well— they beat sixty-six other teams to win the race.

Larimer explains that Posedel, who could run uphill, "would run by us, but the real advantage of having an endurance-riding background is that we had done a number of cross-country races where you have to follow trails marked by ribbons tied around trees. Bill kept getting lost, and we kept passing him when he would get lost. He got lost for twenty or thirty minutes at one point and that's really what enabled us to win."

Since that lucky victory at the ride and tie, Jim Larimer has become a runner as well as an endurance rider. He runs 80 miles per week, training on a portion of the Western States 100-Miler trail. He has been a member of four more victorious ride-and-tie teams—most recently in 1985.

At the 1985 event, Larimer teamed up with Jim Howard, a thirty-year-old forest ranger, who has been a member of two victorious Levi's Ride and Tie teams. Howard also has won two Western States 100-Mile Endurance Runs. On one occasion he won the Western States only six days after winning the Levi's Ride and Tie. On the other occasion he won that ultramarathon just a few days after a second-place finish at the Levi's event. Obviously, Jim Howard recuperates quickly.

The ride and tie is as much a test of strategy and teamwork as endurance—although it certainly qualifies in the endurance category, given the ruggedness of the typical course terrain and the distances usually involved. (The Levi's Ride and Tie distance varies; the first race was 25 miles, but others have been as long as 40 miles.) In order to excel at the sport, the two human teammates must know themselves, each other, and the horse quite intimately. They must be ready to adapt to each other's problems and needs during the race while monitoring their horse's physical condition and keeping track of the competition.

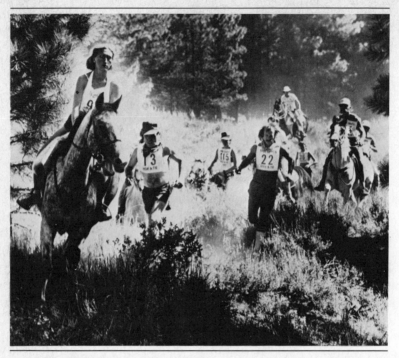

The 1981 Levi's Ride and Tie
COURTESY OF LEVI STRAUSS AND COMPANY

Sometimes ride-and-tie teams opt for short, fast rides, attempting to keep each other in sight as much as possible while maintaining a good tempo. This strategy will work for teams with a very hardy horse and runners who can withstand the punishment of repeated sprints over rough ground. Longer rides make for longer runs for the humans, but that leaves greater rest time for all. The horse gets a longer rest while tied up and waiting for the next rider, and the riders have longer to recuperate from their hikes. And of course some teams opt for a longer run for one partner than the other to accommodate differences in stamina, speed, and experience.

Needless to say, the short-and-fast strategy may backfire, bringing the team to the halfway mark in excellent time, but too depleted to finish the race so fast. Just as bad, going all out can cost the team valuable time waiting at vet checks while the horse recovers enough to continue.

The first Levi's Ride and Tie in 1971 had only two superficial veterinary exams: one before and one during the race. Rigorous vet checks were instituted after two horses died in that first Levi's race. Inexperience, overcompetitiveness, or plain ignorance may blind a person to a horse's limits in a contest, and one competitor approached Bud Johns about the problem. That contestant, Dr. John Steere, a veterinarian, became the head vet for the Levi's race in years that he and his wife D'Ann have not competed. The veterinary procedures Steere instituted have prevented any further fatalities.

Now there are usually four vet checks in a 40-mile race. At each one veterinarians and veterinary students watch the horses trot by, checking for lameness (limping, favoring, or head bobbing are good diagnostics), and they perform hands-on tests. The tests usually include measuring the horse's pulse and respiration rates (P and R's). Horses whose P and R's do not fall below the standard for that particular check point (often 68 or 72 for either) are automatically sidelined ten minutes before being retested, so it's not uncommon to see crews sponging down horses and making their own P and R measurements before turning the horse over to the vet. Other tests vets may make are hydration checks (a well-watered horse's gums will return to normal color after being pressed much faster than when dehydrated) and tests for digestion (productive gut sounds), which ceases when a horse is overly stressed.

The steed of choice for ride and ties, and for endurance riding in general, is an Arabian or an Arabian mix. That breed is preferred because of its excellent endurance characteristics. Arabians take the heat well and are more resistant to dehydration than other horses. Arabians also don't carry the heavy weight of a lot of extra muscle, as does the quarter horse with its round, thick musculature. In short, the Arabian breed has physiological characteristics in common with elite human runners.

Humans are not entirely neglected in a ride-and-tie vet check, although they are not as closely examined as are horses. A good ride-and-tie vet will talk to the human team members to assess their psychological state and will also take note of their apparent physical condition.

One nice feature of the Levi's Ride and Tie is course variety. Levi Strauss always holds the race in a mountainous western setting, but the venue is shifted from year to year. The Levi's Ride and Tie has been staged at Park City, Utah; New Almaden, California; Angels Camp, California; and Sun River, Oregon.

Another nice feature of the race is the prize money. The sponsor underwrites most of the costs of holding the race and returns the entry fees to the top finishers. In 1985, for instance, the top female, male, and mixed teams each received a $3,000 prize, with a $2,000 bonus going to the overall winning team, Jim Larimer and Jim Howard. One interesting consequence of the prize money is that it makes the Levi's Ride and Tie a horse race, and that gives the state agencies that regulate horse racing some say over the race. At one recent Levi's Ride and

Tie, agents of the California Bureau of Animal Health arrived un-announced to run drug tests on the horses. Ride-and-tie competitors are a principled lot, despite the prize money involved; all the horses showed up clean.

MAN VERSUS HORSE

Humans and horses don't always work together, as they do in ride and ties. Sometimes they compete against each other.

In the earliest days of bicycling it was fairly common to match a bicycle against a horse, in order to prove the value of the new form of transportation. Of course, a cyclist can far exceed the speed and stamina of a horse. Even the unwieldy high-wheel bicycles of the turn of the century could outperform a horse. So the real test is on the ground—running—where the human does not have an unfair advantage.

Jim Oury is a forty-nine-year-old heart surgeon. He also is a marathoner, endurance rider, and finisher of both the Ironman Triathlon and Levi's Ride and Tie. In 1980, Oury and his friend Harold Mildenberger of Hamilton, Montana, were sitting around a campfire, swapping tall tales and polishing off a bottle of Jack Daniel's. Mildenberger was bragging about the endurance and speed of his Arabian, Tara. For some crazy reason—perhaps the Tennessee whiskey had something to do with it—Oury, whose best marathon time is 2:51, told Mildenberger that he thought he could outrun a trained Arabian, if the distance were long enough.

A $500 wager resulted in the Mount-and-Man Marathon. The terms of the bet were that Mildenberger could train his horse for six weeks, but he couldn't bring in a ringer. He would have to use a mount already in his herd. Both the horse and the human could have pacers of their own species, and the course would be a mountainous 26-mile loop trail, starting and finishing at the Ravalli County Fairgrounds in Hamilton.

Word about the challenge spread throughout Montana and the betting was heavy; the odds on the two contestants were even. The local cowboys mostly put their money on the horse, and the distance runners at a nearby college mostly bet on the surgeon. On race day several hundred spectators and bettors were there to see that neither competitor took an unfair advantage.

Mildenberger galloped his mount to an early lead and held on to it until he stopped at the halfway point to sponge off the animal. Oury decreased his deficit to about three minutes at that point, but he never got any closer. At 20 miles Oury realized that he could not possibly win unless the horse came up lame. It didn't. Oury's final time was 3:06.03, well off his personal record, but the best he felt he could do that day on the difficult course. The horse beat him by sixteen minutes.

Probably you are thinking that Yiannis Kouros or Carlos Lopes could easily have beaten Mildenberger's Arabian. The horse's time of 2:50 is good but nowhere near the performance of a world-class human runner. Perhaps you would like to find a wealthy rancher who has great pride in his horses, but little knowledge of distance running. Maybe you could act as Alberto Salazar's agent to arrange a big-money wager against the horse. Both sides could put up stakes, and the race could be run on a horse track, with all the gate receipts and TV revenue going to the winner. Ten percent of $500,000 plus side bets wouldn't be bad.

Well, save your money. Thoroughbreds have done the mile in 1:32.2. Sure, a fast human can beat a slow, out-of-shape horse in long-distance events. But a fast horse can beat a slow human at any distance. Fast horses beat experienced runners at Man-vs-Horse, a pair of back-to-back 50-kilometer runs in Prescott, Arizona, during the summer of 1985. What about world-class runners? The key variable is the training of the horse. No human can run 50 miles in a time under 3:15.00, but well-trained endurance horses have done just that. In 1981, Rush Creek Hans, ridden by Boyd Zontelli, set the current course record of 10:46 for the 100-mile Tevis Cup Ride. Jim King's course record for the Western States 100-Miler, which follows roughly the same course as the Tevis, is 14:54.

MUSH, YOU HUSKIES!

In 1867, when the United States bought Alaska from Russia, Nome was little more than a cold beach where American and Russian whalers would occasionally stop to obtain fresh water from nearby Anvil Creek. Nome is on the Alaskan jut of land directly across the Bering Strait from Siberia. The new American owners named that jut of land the Seward Peninsula, in honor of the secretary of state who had negotiated the Alaska purchase. In the late nineteenth century a few Eskimo tribes occupied the Seward Peninsula, which is larger in area than the state of New York, but otherwise it was nearly uninhabited until the end of the nineteenth century.

Despite earlier discoveries of gold in 1866 by Western Union telegrapher Von Bedeleben, and in 1897 by Eskimo Tom Guarick, it wasn't until an 1898 gold strike that the world took notice of Nome. Then three "sourdoughs" coaxed $1,800 worth of gold out of frozen Anvil Creek, panning with water they had melted over a campfire.

That gold strike opened the population floodgates. By the time of the 1900 census, Nome had 12,480 gold-hungry, rambunctious residents. Many of them lived aboard ships in the harbor. During the gold rush, there were occasionally as many as seventy ships at anchor off Nome.

During the days of gold-rush prosperity, railroads were built from Nome to Council City and from Nome to Lanes Landing. Thus, during the summer months it was possible to unload supplies from Seattle at the harbor and transport them to the interior via the railroads. In winter, however, it was a different story. Temperatures can fall to 60 degrees below zero, freezing much of the Norton Sound and closing the port. Snowdrifts often closed down the interior railroads as well. From late December until early March, the lifeline of Nome became a 1,100-mile dog sled trail through the gold-mining town of Iditarod to the ice-free ports of Seward and Anchorage.

Prospecting for precious metals is little more than gambling, so it comes as no surprise that other forms of wagering were also commonplace in Nome during the first decade of the twentieth century. Naturally, the dog sled teams, which were so essential to winter commerce and survival, drew the attention of the gamblers. The sport of dog sled racing was born. In 1908, in the first of a series of annual dog derbies, sleds raced 408 miles across the frozen tundra from Nome to Candle and back. As the new sport developed, a kennel club was founded in Nome. Dogs were bred for the course and the Alaskan husky emerged as a leaner and meaner version of the Siberian husky. In the Dog Derby of 1910, "Ironman" John Johnson mushed a team of huskies to a 74:14.37 course record. Johnson's team averaged a little better than 5.5 miles per hour for the 408-mile race.

Johnson earned the nickname "Ironman" more than half a century before there were triathlons in Hawaii. It is quite appropriate to call a champion musher an ironman. The dogs by no means do all the work. Mushers often run behind their sleds to lighten the load, and they always have their hands full controlling as many as twenty or more dogs. Those dogs have to be fed and cared for. Snow can easily freeze between the pads of a dog's paw, giving a musher the liability of a lame dog. Temperatures that are substantially below zero can freeze the dogs' and mushers' eyelids shut, and frostbite of any exposed skin is always a hazard. Breathing cold air while jogging behind the dog sled can sear the musher's lungs, so the dog driver constantly has to decide whether it is safer to risk pulmonary injury by running or risk exhausting the dogs by riding. In Ironman Johnson's day, usually there was nobody to come to the aid of a musher whose dogs were sick or injured on the trail.

By the time Johnson set his record, the population of Nome had already begun to decline. The 1910 census lists only 2,600 inhabitants, a 79 percent decrease from the previous count. Ownership of the gold claims largely had passed into the hands of well-financed commercial operators, who could afford the machinery to systematically mine the precious ore. The wild days of the Alaskan gold fields were over by 1920.

Thus, in 1925, Dr. Curtis Welch, of the U.S. Health Service, should have been able to cope with the demands for his services. Welch was the only medical doctor that Nome, Alaska, seemed to need. The 1920 decennial census had reported that only 852 people resided in that town. That census had counted only 55,036 people in the entire Alaska Territory, a land area two and a half times the size of Texas.

Then Dr. Welch began to see a few patients complaining of fever and sore throats. Soon some of Welch's patients had inflamed mucous membranes and swelling of the lymph nodes alongside the neck. When Welch saw signs of thin, soft crusts forming over the affected mucous membranes, his worst fears were confirmed. He had a full-scale diphtheria epidemic on his hands.

There suddenly was more to do than any single physician could handle. Welch might have to perform tracheotomies to save some patients, whose breathing could be blocked by the formation of the crust or "pseudomembrane." But blocked breathing passages were only the most immediate problem. Although the infection by the diphtheria baccillus (corynebacterium diphtheriae) does not spread farther than the lymph nodes, it forms lethal toxins that pass into the blood, affecting nerves, the heart, and other tissue. The body produces its own antitoxins to combat diphtheria toxin, but Welch knew that generally would occur too slowly to save most of his patients. Those who were already sick had to be treated with antitoxin.

Diphtheria is a highly contagious disease spread by airborne bacteria. Infection due to coughing and sneezing very likely would spread throughout the small mining community in a matter of days. Since diphtheria had been brought to North America by the white population, the Eskimos had little natural immunity and were particularly vulnerable.

Fortunately, a vaccine and screening method (the Schick test) was available to Welch. When toxins from live diphtheria bacteria are treated with formaldehyde they are made into a harmless toxoid, which can be injected into healthy people so they will be able to produce antitoxins when they are later infected. The Schick test involves injecting tiny amounts of the toxoid beneath the skin to determine if immunization is required. Those people whose skin reacts to the Schick test lack immunity and need the full injection of the toxoid. The only problem was that Nome had only 75,000 units of out-of-date diphtheria toxoid, and the port was competely icebound.

By January 28, there were four diphtheria deaths, twenty-nine diagnosed cases, and at least fifty people known to have been exposed to the infection. There was no direct telephone or telegraph communication to the outside world, ice would keep the harbor closed until March, and there was no passable road or railroad connection. What could be done? George Maynard, the mayor of Nome, declared a quarantine, closed the schools, and pressed all available nurses into service to aid Dr. Welch. An urgent request for 1 million units of antitoxin was sent by radio to Fairbanks, then was relayed by land telegraph to Seward, and finally by underwater cable from Seward to the U.S. Health Service at Seattle.

But how to get the serum to snowbound Nome? Roy Darling, a veteran naval aviator of World War I, stood by to fly a mercy mission to Nome, once the serum had been transported by ship to Seward and then by train to Anchorage. Perhaps one of two dismantled commercial planes in Anchorage could be made airworthy. But there were other problems. On January 30, 1925, the Associated Press reported from Anchorage that "it was impossible to equip men to endure aviation at temperatures averaging 46 below zero, which have prevailed recently in the Yukon valley." Besides, there was no airstrip in Nome. A water landing was impractical, because it would be too dangerous to carry the cargo across the ice that blocked the port, and landing directly on the ice was equally hazardous.

While the problems of airlifting the serum were contemplated, the town of Nome organized a dog sled relay. Leonard Seppala, a champion musher from the dog derbies, raced 650 miles to Nenana with a team of twenty select huskies. When the serum had been forwarded from Anchorage to Nenana by the Alaska Railroad, Seppala's team began the return trek. He carried the precious 20-pound cargo 520 miles over wilderness trails covered with fresh-fallen snow, while the temperatures were far below zero, and no other human was available to assist him. Seppala handed off the serum to a driver named Hammon, who had been dispatched from Nome, 130 miles away, to meet him. Hammon turned around without rest and raced until he met a musher named Olson. Olson carried the cargo to Golovin, where Gunnar Kasson's team took over. Twenty miles outside Nome, Fred Rohn's team was supposed to relieve Kasson, but the rendezvous was frustrated by a howling blizzard. Since the trail was completely whited out by the storm and the hours of daylight are so short during the Arctic winter, Kasson had to navigate by giving his lead dog, Balto, his head. His team ended up pulling two legs of the trek instead of one, but Kasson covered the total of 54 miles in a record time of 7:40, averaging over 7 miles per hour.

Mail service by dog sled on the trail between Nenana and Nome normally required twenty-five days. The record for the trail had been nine days, but the mercy relay of 1925 required only five and a half days. The diphtheria toxoid arrived frozen solid, despite efforts to pack it in insulation. Nonetheless, when the serum was thawed it was usable and the epidemic claimed only five lives. The sled relay saved Nome.

The New York Times published twenty-eight different articles and editorials about the progress of the sled relay, and dog lovers wanted to erect a statue in New York's Central Park to honor Kasson's lead dog, Balto. Every cliché about the friendship between humans and dogs was dusted off; even the United States Senate was not immune to the sentiment. Yet the story of the endurance sled relay that rescued a city was only newsworthy because technological advances were rapidly making such heroic deeds unnecessary. Airplane and highway connections to remote places have steadily improved, and with the invention of the snowmobile even trails across the Alaskan wilderness have become less challenging.

In 1925, the legendary dog mushers still had a crucial role to play in Arctic and Antarctic expeditions, but by the 1970s they were a vanishing breed. By then snowmobile racing, which has a devastatingly negative impact on the wilderness environment, had largely supplanted sled racing. Only a few sprint races, such as the Fur Rendezvous Race in Anchorage, kept the sport alive. Then on a Saturday in March 1973, several hundred yelping huskies stood anxiously at a public square in Anchorage. The excitement of the dogs became unbearable. Finally, one team at a time, the dogs strained against their harnesses as each sled was sent on its way.

A competition had been created to revive the sport of sled racing and commemorate the canine rescue of Nome. Again a historical event provided part of the impetus to organize an endurance event that involved four-legged contestants. The new race was called the Iditarod, to honor the ghost town that in the 1920s had been a lively gold-mining village near the midpoint of the sled trail between Anchorage and Nome.

Since 1973, the Iditarod Trail Dog Sled Race has become an annual event, commencing the first Saturday in March. On an alternating basis, the annual Iditarod starts from either Nome or Anchorage, and covers the entire trail between the two cities. It is the longest sled race in the world. The Iditarod's trail is longer than 1,100 miles, but the race distance is officially advertised as only 1,049 miles—

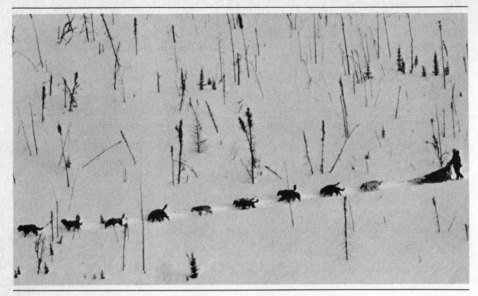

A musher and his team at the 1985 Iditarod Trail
PHOTO BY GREG ANDERSON

because Alaska is the forty-ninth state. Folks do things their own way in Alaska, and what's a few extra miles among friends?

It *is* among friends, too. The Iditarod mushers cooperate during the early portion of the race, because survival on the trail is greatly facilitated by the bunching up of the sixty or seventy teams that enter. The mushers need to work together in order to endure the harsh wilderness conditions of the Iditarod Trail for long periods of time and to break a trail through fresh snow. Twelve days is considered an exceptionally fast race, and seventeen days is nearer the normal time required for the winner to reach Nome. The slower teams may take as much as ten days longer.

Despite the friendliness and cooperation during the early stages of the race, the lead teams *do* compete later. The mushers would like to run their own races, but, apart from one compulsory twenty-four-hour layover, competition demands that they watch each other and get by on two or three hours of sleep each day. In the last 150 miles of the race the contest reaches a fever pitch.

The Iditarod's prizes explain the competitive spirit. In 1985, Libby Riddles, the first musher to reach Nome, carried off $50,000 for her efforts. Alascom, a communications company, gives a $2,000 premium in silver to the first team to reach the halfway point. In all, the first twenty finishers split $200,000.

The investment at risk is great, too. The entry fee is $1,249, and the contestants must pay for the food, veterinary care, and transportation of numerous dogs. (Each team must include a minimum of twelve dogs, and the maximum number allowed is eighteen.) Although few of the dogs hold American Kennel Club papers, the serious mushers breed them specifically for the race, and like good coon dogs in the South, mongrel Alaskan husky pups have been known to go for as much as $6,000. The Iditarod Race Committee has a $1 million annual budget and a full-time, year-round staff to organize the event. These mushers play for high stakes.

Although some mushers have been injured, the difficult and challenging Iditarod has a remarkably good safety record. In the 1985 Iditarod, Colonel Norman Vaughan, an eighty-year-old contestant who had been a musher for Admiral Byrd's 1929 expedition to the South Pole, broke his knee on the trail. But that did not prevent him from signing up for the 1986 race. Thus far, no humans have died in the hazardous race, although there have been a few canine casualties. Precautions are taken to protect the 750 or so dogs in each race, but one or two have died in several of the races.

For instance, 1985 was a year of record snowfall in Alaska, and that made the wild moose herd a hazard to the dogs and their mushers. The large animals sought refuge from the deep snow anywhere there was a clearing. In one twenty-four-hour period twenty moose were killed by collisions with Alaska Railroad trains. Since the Iditarod Race Committee tries to clear its trail with snow-removal machines, in 1985 the contestants encountered many moose. Susan Butcher, who had finished in the money in earlier races and was widely expected to be the first female to win overall, collided with a moose that killed two of her dogs and eliminated her from competition. That left the way clear for Libby Riddles to surprise Iditarod fans by becoming the first female musher to finish number one. In 1986, Butcher finally won.

Apart from occasional accidents, the dogs fare well. During the race, each dog eats about 150 pounds of food, much of which is shipped ahead to the twenty-six checkpoints spaced from 40 to 90 miles apart. Unlike the days when the trail was used commercially, mushers must carry sick or injured dogs to the next checkpoint, rather than leave them to fend for themselves. At the checkpoints, the dogs recover with shelter and veterinary care and are later reunited with their owners. Mushers are disqualified if they arrive at Nome with fewer than half as many dogs as they had when they left Anchorage.

Since the moose problem of 1985, some Iditarod contestants have begun to carry pistols on their sleds. Generally, though, wildlife is rarely a great danger. The bears are still hibernating in March. Although mushers do hear haunting howls in the distance, wolves usually are afraid to approach the dogs. During one Iditarod, a sleeping musher who was camped somewhere between Nikolai and McGrath awoke when he heard a commotion in his campsite. When he looked up, it was into the mugs of three buffalo. But no harm was done.

Although most teams in the Iditarod come from Alaska, the sport has been resurrected on a national—and international—scale. The 1985 Iditarod had mushers from ten countries, as well as the states of Montana, Minnesota, New York, and Michigan. There are at least one hundred North American sled races, mostly at sprint distances shorter than 20 miles. A sanctioning group, the International Sled Dog Racing Association, operates out of Indiana.

In March 1984, twenty-six sled teams competed in the first annual Yukon Quest, a 900-mile race across an international border. The course stretches from Whitehorse, in Canada's Yukon Territory, to Fairbanks, Alaska. Climate inevitably requires the Yukon Quest to compete against the Iditarod for participation. Only the first few weeks of spring are meteorologically suitable for sled racing. Conditions are too severe in the dead of winter, and the snow might be melted later in the season. Even if the events didn't overlap, it's not advisable to race the same dogs twice in one season. Still, the Iditarod Race Committee seems to welcome the competition, seeing emulation as evidence that they have achieved their goal to revive the sport.

UNDER HUMAN POWER

*U*NASSISTED by other animals or machinery, humans are able to travel for relatively long periods of time at speeds approaching 13 miles per hour. Some humans can lift as much as a few hundred pounds. Large numbers of humans working together and using rudimentary tools were able to lift blocks of stone weighing many tons to build the pyramids. Human-powered machines, such as windlasses, bicycles, oared vessels, skis, and blocks and tackle, were later developed to use human power even more effectively and efficiently.

Yet, compared to our ambitions to build great structures and travel at rapid speeds, our muscles have been a puny source of power. By getting beasts of burden, wind, or falling water to provide the power, our early ancestors managed to multiply greatly the speed at which we could move and the amount of work we could do. Gradually scientists, engineers, and inventors learned how to harness the tremendous energy in steam, electricity, and petroleum. Later still, we developed nuclear and solar energy.

Despite all that technological development, a large proportion of the planet's work still is accomplished by human power. This is particularly true in less developed countries. For instance, the foundation for a building can be excavated very rapidly by earth-moving equipment, but throughout much of the world that task is more commonly and more economically accomplished by a human crew of ditch diggers. It's very easy to drive one's automobile to the grocery store, but it often is necessary or more pleasurable to walk or ride a bicycle on such errands. It also is comforting to know that, if energy supplies became unavailable or transit workers go on strike, we can still do work and travel under our own power. Perhaps part of the appeal of endurance sport stems from the subliminal realization that human exertion may become essential at any time.

The earliest endurance sports involved humans running, walking, swimming, or climbing completely under their own power. As machines such as the rowboat and, much later, the bicycle were developed, it was natural for humans to compete in endurance contests using those contrivances. As motors that could replace human power for land vehicles and boats were invented, the old human-powered machines did not completely disappear. The sports involving human power for vehicles did not disappear either, and since fitness has become a worldwide preoccupation those sports have flourished.

Some endurance athletes row racing shells or paddle canoes or kayaks. Others race on skis, ice skates, roller skates, or bicycles. In the past few decades some athletes have been the power source for streamlined human-powered land vehicles, bicycles and tricycles whose fairings and other devices to "cheat" the wind would disqualify them from conventional cycling competition. Less common is the endurance athlete who acts as both the engine and the pilot for human-powered airplanes and blimps.

Some cyclists, rowers, and cross-country skiers claim that their sports are better aerobic exercise than running. Arguably, running is more damaging to joints, bones, and muscles than are the smooth motions of rowing, skiing, or bicycling. Rowers and skiers also point to the fact that, unlike running, their sports exert the upper body as well as the legs. Runners rebut by pointing out that their sport requires very little equipment and can be done virtually anywhere. You can run in place in a prison cell, but just try cross-country skiing in Oklahoma during the summer. Cross-country skiing fanatics respond that they use "roller-skis" during the summer. The debate over which aerobic exercise is best will never be settled, but certainly the individual level of effort makes a difference in how strenuous the activity is.

For the most part, machines, such as bicycles or rowboats, and tools, such as skis, enable humans to move much more rapidly across the land or water than they could without mechanical assistance. Similarly, those human engines can cover much greater distances than unmechanized runners, swimmers, or walkers. The human-powered machines provide practical transportation for almost anybody, and athletes can respond to the mechanical advantage by maintaining the exertion level of runners and swimmers and simply accomplishing more.

Endurance athletes often are competitive or curious about their personal performance boundaries, and various races exist to test the mettle of bicyclists, rowers, canoers, kayakers, and cross-country skiers. Recently a few prizes have inspired unprecedented endurance achievement in human-powered aviation. Here are a few of the endurance events in which the contestants are the power plant for a machine.

YO HO, HEAVE, HO

Every schoolchild in America used to learn that Christopher Columbus discovered America in 1492. Of course, that lesson neglected two
facts. First, there were upwards of 2 million Indians already here when
Columbus "discovered" America. And second, other Europeans had
visited America almost five hundred years earlier than Columbus.
Those earlier explorers were Norsemen, and they came here by rowboat.

Centuries before the Scandinavian sailors first rowed oared galleys, the ancient Greeks, Persians, and Romans had already built great
warships that were propelled by oars. In the fifth century B.C., Greek
city-states launched human-powered ships, which were 115 feet long
by 11.5 feet wide. (Later oared galleys were even larger than that.)
One hundred and seventy rowers provided the power for these Greek
boats, which are called triremes because the oarsmen were arranged
in three vertical tiers. (Biremes with two banks of oars were also built,
as were quadriremes with four rowers and quinquiremes with five
rowers per station.) Writing in the April 1981 issue of *Scientific American*, Vernard Foley and Werner Soedel speculated that triremes could
attain speeds greater than 11.5 knots. According to Foley and Soedel,
triremes may have been light and fast enough to permit semiplaning
like modern speedboats, which means triremes may have reached ve-
locities as great as 17 knots! That speed would compare very favorably
to the records for modern eight-oared shells. The 2,000-meter record
for still-water rowing (13.46 miles per hour) was last set in 1976 by an
East German crew at the Montreal Olympics on a 2,000-meter course.
Triremes were built for speed, because their principal offensive tactic
was to ram the enemy.

Foley and Soedel argue that, contrary to common belief, the rowers of the triremes were almost certainly not slaves, but were highly
paid patriotic freemen. A disgruntled galley slave, rebelling against
the lash, could completely disrupt forward progress by fouling an oar
or simply pulling out of sequence. Rowing triremes required a great
deal of teamwork, and the rowers were skilled endurance athletes, not
shackled and beleaguered slaves.

Just as they do now on modern racing shells, coxswains probably
called out the rhythm of the stroke in order to keep the rowers in
synchrony. That measure was essential, because coordinating the rowing was a difficult requirement for sailing the multioared warships.
That problem must have reached an extreme several centuries after
the trireme was developed, when Ptolemy IV built a gargantuan catamaran, with an aircraft-carrier-style flat deck connecting the twin

hulls. The catamaran carried artillery in the form of catapults, and one was known to have transported nearly 3,000 marines at one time. The power plant for this "rowboat" was 4,000 oarsmen.

A mercy mission by an Athenian trireme—one of the "small" vessels with *only* 160 oarsmen—provides one of the earliest documented examples of rowers rising to an endurance challenge. In 425 B.C. the city of Mitylene on the island of Lesbos failed in a revolt against its Athenian overlords. At the urging of Cleon, a bloodthirsty Greek orator, Athens' assembly dispatched a trireme to instruct their garrison to put all the citizens of rebellious Mitylene to death. By the next day a more moderate point of view prevailed in the Athenian assembly, and a second trireme was sent to rescind the previous order. The crew of the earlier boat had a twenty-four-hour head start, but they were not in any great rush to deliver their grisly tidings. On the other hand, the second boat's crew, with its message of clemency, rowed continuously at top speed for twenty-four hours, fueled by rice cakes soaked in wine, which the oarsmen reportedly ate while they were rowing. Averaging 9 knots, the second boat covered the 214 miles to Mitylene in roughly half the time of the earlier boat. The first boat had arrived shortly ahead of the second vessel, but fortunately the stay of execution was delivered before the genocide could be carried out.

Gradually sails and steam replaced human sinew as the motive force for oceangoing vessels. On the practical side, the rowboat and canoe were retained for short trips and conveying cargo and passengers from a large ship to shore. On the recreational side, rowing, canoeing, and kayaking have survived as sports.

Unlike the ancient craft, modern racing shells are slender and light and usually require one to eight rowers. The larger modern shells are similar to their huge predecessors in that they carry a coxswain.

Paddling

Rowers distinguish themselves from canoers and kayakers in that they look where they have already been rather than where they are going. Canoers and kayakers look forward, working the paddle by a push-pull motion of the arms, whereas the rower pulls with both arms simultaneously.

Ancient Eskimos, who stretched hides over lightweight frames to make covered canoes, get credit for inventing the kayak. The modern kayak may be made from various materials, including canvas, wood, and plastic. To propel their boats, skilled kayakers gracefully crank their double-bladed paddles in a circular motion that dips first one blade, then the other. When a novice tries the motion it sometimes looks like a drunkard trying to eat soup with a spoon that has bowls

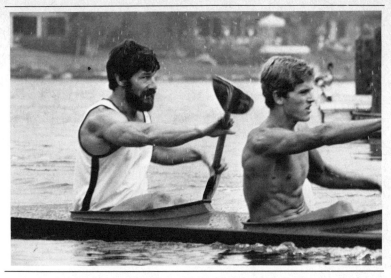

A double kayak at West Lake, California.

PHOTO BY BUDD SYMES

on each end. Kayaking takes some training and physical coordination. In particular, novices have to learn how to right themselves without panicking when a kayak rolls over.

Kayaking and canoeing are popular sports in the United States and Canada, possibly because the sleek canoe designs developed by American Indians were imitated by white settlers, who gave those boats an important role in this continent's pioneer history. Paddling a canoe across a lake or down a rapid stream, it's easy to feel connected to early American fur traders or explorers such as Lewis and Clark.

In the book *Canoe Racing*, Fred Heese says, "the first canoe race was held when the second canoe was built." Canoeing is an Olympic sport, and there are numerous amateur and professional races held throughout North America. There are flat-water canoe races, white-water competitions for the adventurous, and marathon canoe races ideal for the endurance athlete.*

The Texas Water Safari, a major endurance canoeing event, is a 419-mile race down the San Marcos and Guadalupe rivers. It requires canoeists to brave rapids, to portage around numerous logjams and obstacles, to endure the sweltering temperatures of Texas in early June, and to fight the choppy waves of San Antonio Bay, where the event

---

Canoe Racing, by Fred Heese, includes names and addresses of race directors who can give you information about canoeing and kayaking events. You might also seek race information from the American Canoe Association (7217 Lockport Place, Lorton, Virginia 22079) or from *Canoe* magazine. (See list of periodicals for address.)

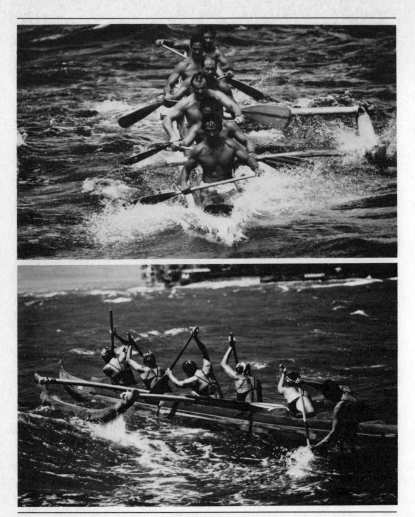

*These Hawaiian outrigger canoeists seem oblivious to
the choppiness of the Kawai Channel.*

PHOTO BY MONTE COSTA

finishes. A very respectable finish for that event, which allows for no
sleep and little rest, is about thirty-seven hours.

In Hawaii, numerous races and regattas for the long oceangoing
canoes inspire many endurance athletes to stay in training. For instance, each fall since 1952, paddlers have raced their sleek outrigger
canoes 40.1 miles across Kawai Channel between Molokai and Oahu.
Some years that stretch of ocean water has been extremely rough. The
race, which is called the Molokai Ho'e (Molokai paddle), attracts an
international field of about forty-five six-man canoes. Since 1975, about
twenty canoes have paddled the same course in a separate women's
race, the Na Wahine O Ko Kai, which means women of the sea. The

paddlers must average a back-breaking pace of about 6 knots for five or six hours to win these races. The Outrigger Canoe Club has been a perennial favorite in both the men's and women's races, frequently beating teams from the mainland, Polynesia, and Japan. Membership in the Outrigger Canoe Club confers considerable status in Hawaiian society.

Rowing

By A.D. 1300, the canals of Venice already had been the venue for a rowing regatta. On August 1, 1716, a sculling race occurred on the Thames between London Bridge and Chelsea. Known as the Doggett's Coat and Badge, that crew race is still staged each year.

In many countries, rowing is mostly a club sport. However, since the beginning of the twentieth century, crew racing has been largely an intercollegiate sport in the United States, Canada, and Great Britain. The first intercollegiate sporting event of any sort in America was an 1852 race in which four crews from Harvard and Yale met on New Hampshire's Lake Winnipesaukee. Although the form of the race has evolved over the years, the Harvard-Yale matchup is still a tradition-steeped annual event. Staged during a two-week period after exams, the Harvard-Yale race is surrounded by shenanigans reminiscent of an extended panty raid. Oh, those college boys!

Many fans of crew would be surprised to learn that during the last half of the nineteenth century rowing in singles was a thriving professional sport. Lots of money changed hands as the result of heavily promoted, well-attended rowing contests. Like other professional sports during that era, rowing eventually fell victim to its own chicanery and excesses. The amateur movement, with its upper-class biases, was sweeping through athletics, and the public grew weary of the gambling, cheating, and sabotaging of boats that characterized professional rowing. By the time collegiate rowing came on the scene, the professionals had been thoroughly discredited. It was considered scandalous to have the old pros even coach the gentlemen collegiate rowers, and consequently their knowledge of legitimate techniques was lost. The early collegiate rowers often rowed badly because the pros were excluded from coaching.

While rowing clubs in such solidly midwestern venues as Detroit have long and illustrious histories, collegiate rowing still carries many of the snobbish connotations of the eastern old-school tie. Now regattas are cropping up in such unlikely places as San Diego, California. Early in the spring, when the ice is still breaking up on some northern rivers, the San Diego Crew Classic requires Ivy League rowers to associate with teams from such plebeian schools as the University of California and the University of Washington. The bloodline has thinned so greatly that there also are Southern Intercollegiate Rowing Association and Pac-10 regattas.

Some good old girls also have elbowed their way into the crew-jock network. Those women sweat, too; they don't just glisten.

Even Ohio has gotten into the act. In 1982, Cincinnati attorney Bill Engeman, who rowed for Brown in the early 1960s, promoted a national collegiate regatta on a man-made lake in the midst of Ohio farmland. Winning teams from major regional races were invited to attend, and the event sponsors picked up the tab for their travel. The race is now an annual event, and the crew that wins this de facto national championship represents the United States in England's prestigious Henley Regatta. (At the Henley Regatta the Yankees must race at what is called "Henley distance," 2,112 meters instead of the 2,000 meters to which they are accustomed.)

Increasingly in America, rowing has become popular outside of academe, with rowing clubs springing up on rivers and bays across the country.* As of 1985, 340 organizations were affiliated with the U.S. Rowing Association, and of late the number of groups has grown by 10 percent each year.

One explanation for the recent renaissance of sculling is the development of relatively stable, individual and tandem training shells, such as the Alden and the Laser. Made of plastic, they are much easier to operate than traditional racing shells. Even expert rowers can admit without embarrassment that they occasionally tip over. Compared to the slender, wooden shells, the training boats have broad bottoms that resist capsizing.

Another reason the use of training shells has increased the popularity of rowing is that mass-produced plastic shells are less expensive than many of their elegant, handmade, wooden forebears. In the last few years shell manufacturers also have produced racing models made from exotic synthetic materials, such as carbon fibers and Dupont Kevlar. These high-tech boats are stiff and responsive. Like the fiberglass pole for high jumping, they offer a competitive advantage. Unlike synthetic training boats, the new plastic racing boats are more expensive than the classic wooden shells.

The majority of rowing events are only 2,000 meters long. (Women previously raced 1,000 meters, but now they usually also compete at 2,000 meters.) It is common, however, to row a great deal farther in

*Local rowing organizations and events can be located by consulting the U.S. Rowing Association and its magazine, Rowing USA. The address for both the publication and the organization is 251 North Illinois Street, Suite 980, Indianapolis, Indiana 46204.

practice. There also is a recent trend toward promotion of some longer rowing events. Two- to four-mile *head* races (which usually begin at the headwaters of a river) have become popular on rivers and bays throughout America. The distances for head races vary according to the length of navigable water available. Peggy O'Neal, of the U.S. Rowing Association, says, "Everybody likes head races in the fall, because that's when they're working on their endurance; then in the spring they switch over to the 2,000-meter races." Head races are typically time trials, where the race is against the clock rather than other boats. That format permits a much larger number of boats to participate than could normally fit across most rivers. It also allows spectators to see almost constant action.

The Boston Marathon of rowing is the Head-of-the-Charles Regatta in Cambridge, Massachusetts. That event, which was dreamed up in 1966 by insurance executive D'Arcy McMahon and two of his rowing buddies, boasts greater participation than any other single-day event in rowing. The Cambridge regatta was the first head race, and it handles as many rowers as possible, limiting each heat to forty boats. Over two thousand rowers participate in men's and women's divisions for singles, doubles, fours, and eights. Enthusiastic spectators line 3 miles of the Charles River to watch the event.

The Head-of-the-Charles is structured to encourage participation by all sorts of rowers. There are "schoolboy" classes for rowers under nineteen and a half years old, and three masters classes, for thirty to thirty-nine, forty to forty-nine, and fifty-plus-year-old rowers. Lightweight male crews, whose average weight is under 160 pounds, have a separate class, as do females who weigh less than 130 pounds.

The Head-of-the-Charles has been the inspiration for numerous other head races, such as the Head-of-the-Hooch, a race on the Chattahoochee River in Georgia. The Head-of-the-Mississippi, Head-of-the-Des Moines, Head-of-the-Tennessee, and Head-of-the-Schuylkill are just a few of the other head races.

Since 1982, the Sound Rowers, a club that plies the waters of Puget Sound, has sponsored an annual marathon row around Bainbridge Island. The course is 23.2 nautical miles. (That's 26.7 miles to landlubbers.) A shorter "cruising course" race of 11 nautical miles (12.2 miles) is staged at the same time. For the marathon event, times are reported separately for each of four classes: double shells and wherries, single shells and wherries, single kayaks, and canoes. (A wherry is loosely defined as a training single.)

Competition has improved performance for the circumnavigation of Bainbridge Island. After Alex Kimball and Christine Hall won the 1984 event, the *Sound Rower's Newsletter* speculated, "With all the

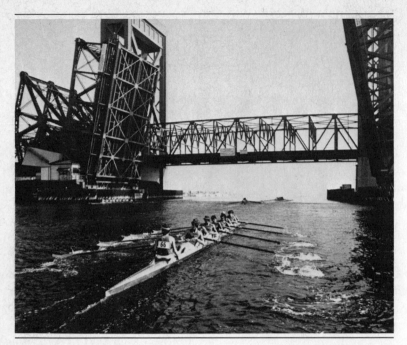

The Head of the Harbor rowing regatta, Los Angeles Harbor. PHOTO BY BUDD SYMES

data in, it appears Bainbridge Island has gotten smaller since the first marathon; how else to explain Kimball's '82 time of 6 hours in his Catalina Wherry, 4 hours 50 minutes in '83 in a 17' Graham shell, and this year's 11 boats finishing in under 4 hours 45 minutes?" Kimball and Hall averaged 5.67 knots for the marathon.

In 1976 Charles Hathaway, president of the Los Angeles Athletic Club, decided to celebrate his birthday by rowing the 37 miles of open ocean from California's Catalina Island to Marina Del Rey. Why not? The course is over 50 kilometers, and it was Hathaway's fiftieth birthday. Charlie's son, Steve, is manager of the California Yacht Club, and that organization has perpetuated the birthday row as the Great California Yacht Club Catalina to Marina Del Rey Rowing and Paddling Derby. The yacht club bills its event as the ultramarathon of rowing, and over the years has held it in weather conditions that *Rowing USA* describes as varying "from flat calm to very rough and windy." A team consisting of John Aranson and Rob Jackson rowed a double to a 5:21.46 overall victory in the October 7, 1984, race.

Winter can be a tough time for many crew jocks because the weather prohibits getting out on the water. Many of them compensate by practicing other endurance sports (e.g., cross-country skiing) and by workouts on machines called rowing ergometers. Along with being about as inspiring as breaking rocks in solitary confinement, rowing

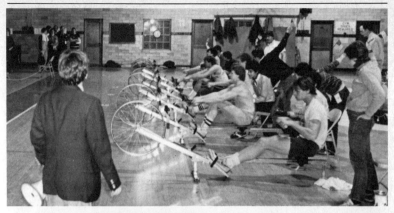

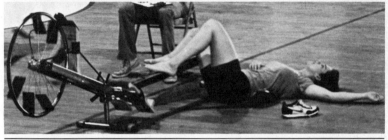

TOP: *The CRASH-B sprints*   COURTESY CONCEPT II, INC.

BOTTOM: *Ann Strayer recovers from a CRASH-B sprint.*
COURTESY OF CONCEPT II, INC.

an ergometer is not quite the same as the "real thing." It's difficult for a machine to replicate the feel of pulling a boat through water; in particular, the glide portion of the stroke is missing.

Nonetheless, technology often provides an answer. A few manufacturers have come out with ergometers that imitate the real thing pretty well. The Concept II is one brand of "natural-feeling" ergometer highly regarded by rowers. It nicely simulates the glide portion of the stroke. You can even hook the Concept II to home computers, so you can watch yourself on a video display rowing against an imaginary competitor. But every pop sociologist knows that videogames promote rather than reduce isolation. So, the old-school tie and camaraderie of the boathouse are still missing.

Lately, however, the Concept II has spawned a new endurance sport, indoor rowing championships, which provide the missing companionship. In Boston, Tiff Wood has promoted CRASH-B Sprints, indoor rowing contests on Concept II machines. (Wood distinguished himself on Harvard and Olympic teams, and CRASH-B is an acronym for Charles River All-Star Has Beens.) Shifts of rowers perform 5-mile "pieces" on the machine, with the semifinal victory going to the six rowers who register 5 miles on their odometers in the least time. The six finalists then compete in the same heat for the overall title.

In February 1985, the winning men's time was sculling star Andy Sudduth's 7:56.3. Jeanne Flanagan won the women's competition with a time of 9:01.1. If you want to accelerate your heartbeat, just try to row that fast sometime. If you succeed, you should be able to nail a medal or two in an upcoming Olympics, just as Sudduth and Flanagan did in 1984.

Wood and his cronies started the CRASH-B in 1982, and by 1985 participation in the competition had grown to more than six hundred rowers. Throughout the United States, in places like Florida, Wisconsin, Washington, D.C., and the state of Washington, CRASH-B races have been staged. Just set up a few machines in a large, well-ventilated gymnasium and hundreds of hibernating rowers will crawl out of their winter holes to contribute buckets of sweat to a CRASH-B event.

It is common for endurance athletes to seek out or try to concoct events that are the longest in the world for their sports. Rowers are no exception. Sometimes these efforts at one-upmanship succeed; sometimes they backfire. In the fall of 1983, the Rochester University Crew Club raised $1,000 for new equipment by soliciting pledges for a 55-mile "row-a-thon" down the Barge Canal from Lockport to Rochester, New York. (The Barge Canal includes sections of the historic Erie Canal.) When the city of Rochester asked the university to produce an activity for the city's sesquicentennial celebration, Gary Stockman, a coach and founding member of the crew club who also works in the university's public relations department, suggested repeating the previous fall's row-a-thon as a race. The idea was to bill the 55-mile event as the world's longest crew race. The city of Rochester readily accepted the university's proposal, but there was only one problem: Stockman discovered that the *Guinness Book of Records* listed a 96-mile Swiss race, the Tour du Lac Leman, as the longest crew event. The solution: double the course. Row 55 miles from Lockport to Rochester, and then row back, making their own race 14 miles longer than the Swiss event.

The Rochester Club mailed invitations to every crew club in America, and received expressions of interest from fifteen teams. When race day arrived, August 19, 1984, only four boats actually entered the water: the Rochester boat—with Stockman on board—the Union College boat, the Topeka Rowing Club's boat from Kansas, and the LSD Rowing Club's boat. (LSD stands for Long Slow Distance, and that club was an ad-hoc female crew whose members came from New England, California, and Rochester.)

Weather during the race included rain, hot sun, clouds, and wind.

Race rules included a mandatory five-minute rest period at the Spencer Lift Bridge, but otherwise doing well required continuous effort. For instance, the Rochester rowers took their breakfast break in pairs, as the other six members of their crew continued to row. The preferred technique for passing under lift bridges, which often are just inches above the water, is to do what the Rochester Crew called a "sun drill." When the coxswain yells, "Sun drill," each rower leans back onto the knees of the next rower and the bridge passes just above their noses as the boat glides through. Stopping for the bridge to lift is too time-consuming.

Unfortunately, the "world's longest" crew race fell short of its promise. Because of a stronger than anticipated current in the canal, it took ten hours and three minutes for the first crew (Rochester) to reach the turnaround, several hours longer than predicted. Race officials realized that the canal's lift bridges would close at 11:00 P.M., and though the shells would be able to get under the bridges, the support boats were too big to follow. To avoid the danger of unsupported nighttime rowing, the race was called at the 55-mile point. The 96-mile Tour du Lac Leman retains its distinction as the longest race.

Transoceanic Rowing

Boat races of up to 96 miles are formidable, but Kathleen and Curtis Saville might consider them merely warmups. Between March 18 and June 10, 1981, the Savilles rowed their oceangoing craft, the *Excalibur*, from Casablanca, Morocco, to English Harbor, Antigua, a 3,000-nautical-mile jump across the Atlantic Ocean.

Both Curtis and Kathleen shared an interest in rowing when they met at the Narragansett Boat Club in Providence, Rhode Island. Kathleen had rowed crew as captain of her college team, and Curtis first considered the transatlantic adventure after he survived a bad storm while replicating Henry David Thoreau's canoe trip across a Maine lake. In the October 1981 issue of *Smithsonian*, the Savilles wrote, "When we returned from a trip together on Moosehead Lake in an oar-rigged canoe in 1979, we took two momentous steps: we got married and started to think seriously about a transatlantic row."

The Savilles were not the first transatlantic rowers. Way back in 1897, Frank Samuelson and George Harbo set a record of fifty-five days for a 3,075-mile crossing from New York to England. Another recent transatlantic crossing by Gerard d'Aboville was made arduous by five capsizings, but ultimately he was successful, too. A pair that rowed the *Puffin* out of Virginia in 1966 was less fortunate in an attempt to reach England. The *Puffin* was found drifting off Newfoundland, but no clue to the fate of its crew was found.

Curtis and Kathleen Saville made diligent preparations to avoid the same fate. They sought the advice of Ed Montesi, a boat designer who had rowed on the U.S. team at the 1959 Pan American Games. With Montesi's help they came up with a boat custom-designed for Atlantic crossings; it had a covered cabin and was twenty-five feet, two inches long and five feet, three inches across the beam. The hull was to be a molded sandwich of fiberglass mat and cloth layers around half-inch-thick airex foam. Featuring waterproof compartments, the *Excalibur* was designed to resist sinking. Weight was distributed so that the boat would be self-righting if it flipped over. As they consumed the 95 gallons of freshwater in their bottles, the boat would rise, permitting faster rowing, but they could always refill the empties with seawater, sacrificing speed for stability in the event of a storm.

Friends from the Narragansett Boat Club helped the Savilles build their craft in a Touisset, Rhode Island, barn. Construction required seven months. When the hull was ready, the Savilles experimented with the ideal position for oars by moving temporarily mounted Martin Marine Oarmasters—systems of portable oarlocks and sliding seats— into several locations. After their research on the ideal rowing position, they built permanent oar stations in the uncovered area of the central deck. *Excalibur* was empowered by two pairs of sculling oars similar to those used on shells. The boat had two adjustable daggerboards to manipulate steering, but they also equipped the boat with an electronic autopilot, which would allow them to keep their vessel on course without having to consider how hard they were rowing on a particular side. To charge the batteries that would power their autopilot, as well as their radio and lights for navigation and illumination, they installed solar cells on the cabin top. Much of the equipment was donated by manufacturers.

During the construction period, the Savilles conditioned their bodies for the upcoming ordeal by running 5 miles per day, rowing, and pumping iron. As soon as the boat was seaworthy, they conducted 200 miles of shakedown cruises to get used to their vessel and further build their rowing muscles.

When all was in readiness, the Savilles transported their boat to Casablanca aboard a Yugoslavian freighter. They had their first opportunity to row in heavy seas right after leaving Casablanca. The storm hit them before they even had their sea legs. Their plan had been to sprint away from the African coast, to escape the possibility of violently running aground and being crushed against rocks. Wretchedly seasick, they alternated leaning over the side to throw up. During this stormy period of the voyage the Savilles wore their safety harnesses even inside the cabin, in case their boat was swamped by waves, which they described as "Matterhorn-shaped mountains" that came at them from two directions simultaneously. The gale made their rowing even more difficult than normal, which is going some. They described their situation in the January 1982 issue of *Oarsman*: "Pulling the combined weight of the boat and supplies (nearly a ton) caused a lot of strain on our bodies . . . Blisters popped, stung in the salt water and showed signs of infection. The best we could do was put on iodine and tape. We tried rowing with gloves but didn't like the loss of control."

After four days, they were able to obtain a celestial fix on their position. Just trying to stay steady to use the sextant for a sun sight in the rolling and pitching boat became a recurring ordeal of the voyage. During the storm they had been pulled 100 miles south and had only cleared the African coast by a few miles. Worse yet, they had drifted into a war zone, the waters off Sidi Ifni, where Morocco and Mauritania were contesting ownership of the Spanish Sahara. They were forced to take their radar reflector off their mast and douse their navigational lights to keep from being discovered and sunk by either combatant's naval forces.

Political turmoil and drug traffic lately has made life at sea in a small boat a risky proposition. Piracy on the high seas is commonplace. The Savilles turned west and rowed long hours to clear the dangerous war zone, but nonetheless were later frightened by an unidentified trawler that showed more interest in them than is common in that area of the ocean. Perhaps the flare gun that Curt brandished seemed a more substantial weapon than it actually was, because eventually the threatening trawler turned away from the *Excalibur*.

After twenty-four days, the weary rowers reached the Canary Islands, where on Tenerife they repaired the badly corroded wiring to their solar panels. The electrical equipment was essential to the operation of their autopilot. Their respite on land lasted ten days, then they resumed their journey, entering an easterly current system. For about two weeks they enjoyed a calm ocean and the knowledge that the currents were helping rather than hindering their progress across the Atlantic. They enjoyed this part of their voyage and even supplemented their diet with gifts from the ocean—flying fish that landed on the *Excalibur* of their own volition. Then they heard an ominous radio report about the birth of tropical storm Arlene.

Spurred on by fear of Arlene, which prematurely inaugurated the hurricane season of 1981, the Savilles turned their crossing into a race and took five days off Samuelson and Harbo's 55-day record. To do this they rowed seven to eight hours a day, either simultaneously or in shifts. As the seas kicked up, they learned to stroke rapidly up one side of a huge wave and then raise their oars to surf down the other side. During these maneuvers their autopilot kept them basically on

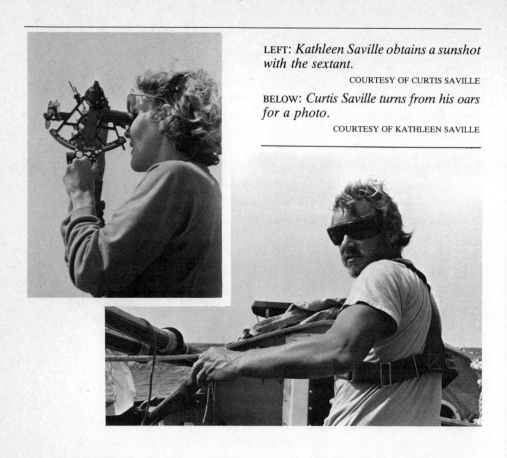

LEFT: *Kathleen Saville obtains a sunshot with the sextant.*

COURTESY OF CURTIS SAVILLE

BELOW: *Curtis Saville turns from his oars for a photo.*

COURTESY OF KATHLEEN SAVILLE

Landfall at Queensland, Australia, after 10,000 miles of rowing.

COURTESY OF KATHLEEN SAVILLE

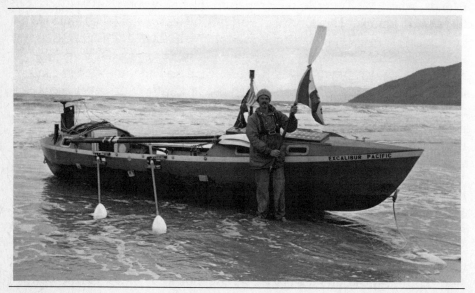

course. By "surfing" they briefly were able to achieve exhilarating speeds approaching 6 knots.

The increased rowing made their bodies hurt during waking hours and turned their dreams into bizarre explanations of their aches and pains. One time Curt dreamed that a sheep, which had been conjured by a medium, bit him on the neck. Then he awoke to severe shoulder and neck pain; their hard rowing to escape the storm had aggravated an old injury. The rush of water began to sound like human voices to them, and they actually searched the boat for a dog, whose barking they had imagined. They conducted disjointed conversations that would drop in midsentence and then be completed days later. But they managed to outrun the storm, arriving ahead of schedule at an approximate midpoint, longitude 40 degrees west. Then they had to fight easterly storm systems, which hovered around the approaches to the Caribbean Sea.

Eighty-four days after they left Casablanca they finally caught sight of their destination—the cliffs known as the Gates of Hercules, at the entrance to Antigua's English Harbor. As they approached the treacherous opening to the harbor, local yachtsmen watched them from high cliffs and radioed valuable piloting assistance. To pull through the adverse currents and make it around the deadly reefs, the Savilles had to do "power pieces"—rapid sets of strong strokes. Finally, they made it into port.

Later the Savilles wrote, "We were sad in a way, to see our private world of rowing and living on the Atlantic come to an end." Just to keep their oars in the water, in 1984 Curt and Kathleen left Lima, Peru, on a rowboat trip to Cairns, Australia. They wanted to be the first rowers to cross the Pacific. Their trip covered approximately 10,000 miles.

For this trip they added one pair of sweep oars to their sculling oars. Because sweep oars are the type used on eight-person crew shells, this enabled them to row with one hand or two if they experienced any injury, such as Curt's sore shoulder.

They followed the Humboldt-Current route that Thor Heyerdahl used for part of his journey on the sailing raft *Kon-Tiki*. The Savilles accomplished the biggest jump of their new journey when they reached the Marquesas Islands in October 1984. After a five-month layover for the hurricane season, they left the Marquesas for American Samoa. Then they rowed to Vanuatu (formerly the New Hebrides). Finally, they proceeded directly to the Great Barrier Reef outside Cairns, Australia.

Peter Bird, who in 1982 attempted a similar voyage from San Francisco, fell just 60 miles short of his final destination. He crashed his boat against the Great Barrier Reef and had to call the Australian navy for assistance. His rowboat was lost completely when it swamped and sank during the towing, but he survived. The Savilles checked and rechecked their navigation to avoid Bird's fate as they passed through the reef. But, before they got there, they turned over in a storm. Fortunately, the *Excalibur* is self-righting, and they were able to complete their voyage in their own boat.

LEGGINGS OF BIRCHBARK

In America, the popularity of cross-country (Nordic) skiing is a relatively recent phenomenon. Although the legendary Snowshoe Thompson reportedly skied the U.S. mail across the Sierra Nevadas as early as 1856, very few Americans did any cross-country skiing prior to 1970. America fielded Olympic teams in the sport, but there were relatively few recreational cross-country skiers back then. There were some notable exceptions, such as 110-year-old Herman "Jackrabbit" Johanssen, who first skied at two years old and still skied a kilometer every day during the winter of his 108th year. However, before 1970 the preponderance of American skiing was Alpine (downhill) rather than Nordic.

Even Johanssen brought his cross-country skiing with him from his native Norway, where he was born in 1875. Before emigrating to the United States, he came to Canada in 1902 to sell railroad equipment and skied much of the route that became the Canadian National Railroad, often in the company of Cree Indians on snowshoes, who gave him the nickname "Jackrabbit." Johanssen plans to set the most basic endurance record of them all: the longevity record. He may make it; he retains his wit and faculties, and doesn't look a day over one hundred.

Alpine skiers take a lift, towbar, tramway, or even helicopter up a hill, and then they glide effortlessly down. Depending on their skill and nerve, Alpine skiers either experience exhilarating trips down the slope or excruciating injuries that threaten life and limb. Orthopedists with good business sense pray for snow. Although downhill skiing requires considerable strength and remarkable agility, many Nordic advocates deride Alpine skiing because it provides much less cardiovascular exercise than does skiing cross-country. It exercises only patience and elbows, they say: patience waiting in the lift lines, and elbows hoisting drinks at the ski lodge bar.

You must climb the hills and traverse the flatlands—as well as race down the hills—to cover terrain on cross-country skis. Without question, skiing cross-country gives an athlete a vigorous aerobic workout, and that brand of skiing has become increasingly popular since 1970, as other endurance sports have experienced similar growth.

Scandinavian Classics

Unlike people in other parts of the world, Scandinavians have strapped on cross-country skis for many centuries. In Sweden, Norway, and Finland cross-country skiing is a way of life; it provides transportation as well as recreation. Since Scandinavia gave the rest of the world cross-country skiing, the sport is often called Nordic skiing. (Downhill skiing evolved in the mountainous regions of Switzerland and Austria, hence the term Alpine skiing.)

To the Nordic people, cross-country skiing has many historical as well as practical connotations. Soldiers who have fought for Scandinavian countries often did so on skis. As recently as the winter of 1939–40, soldiers on cross-country skis defended Finland against invasion by its numerically superior neighbor the Soviet Union. The Russians had expected to overrun Finland in a few days, but ski patrols kept the Red Army pinned down for an entire winter. Although the Finnish defense was not entirely successful, the stubborn resistance of the skiing troops ultimately forced the Soviet Union to concede a large measure of autonomy to Finland.

But sagas of Scandinavian knights errant mounted on skis predate the war between Russia and Finland by more than four hundred years. According to legend, in 1520 a nobleman, Gustav Wasa, tried to arouse the Swedish peasantry near the town of Mora to revolt against the Danes then occupying part of Sweden. Initially, the Swedes did not respond to Gustav's call for rebellion. Later, the people of Mora decided to cast out the Danes, but Gustav, fearing he would be killed, as his father had been in Stockholm, already had fled. Mora dispatched two of its fastest skiers to retrieve Gustav, who had reached the town of Sälen on the Norwegian border. Gustav returned and led a successful insurrection by the Swedes. Subsequently, he was crowned King Gustav Wasa, and his descendants sat on the throne of Sweden until 1654.

In 1922, the quadricentennial of the revolt against Denmark, an annual cross-country ski race was founded to commemorate the ski trip that retrieved Gustav Wasa. The Vasaloppet is staged the first Sunday in March. (*Loppet* means race in Swedish.) That 89-kilometer (55-mile) event from the village of Berga (near Sälen) to Mora now draws more than twelve thousand contestants.* So many applicants have to be turned away from the Vasaloppet that a second race, Öpet Spår (open course), was created to take the overflow. About nine thousand skiers take on the Öpet Spår about one week prior to the

---

*Throughout this book, race distances are reported in the measurement system used by promoters of the race. Occasionally, a metric distance is followed by the English dimension, which is more familiar to American readers. Using both systems of measurement may cause some initial confusion, but you can always convert the distance with the following equation: 1 mile = .621 kilometer.

Vasaloppet. In Scandinavia, cross-country skiing is an endurance sport, attracting as much participation as running does in the United States.

In 1932, Norwegian cross-country skiers founded the Birkebeiner-Rennet, a 55-kilometer (34-mile) event starting in Lillehammer, Norway. This race also traces a historic route used by legendary ski heroes. During the Norwegian civil war of 1206, Skjervald Skrukka and Torstein Skevla, Viking soldiers loyal to King Sverre, skied 55 kilometers to rescue the infant prince Haakon Haakonsson. The Viking skiers carried a payload, young Prince Haakon, and skiers in the modern Birkebeiner-Rennet are required to carry a 12-pound backpack. The birchbark leggings, which those two Vikings wore, are called birke-beiners in Norwegian, and that explains the origin of the name for this *rennet*, or race.

The American Birkebeiner

Tony Wise, an American veteran of World War II with a Harvard MBA, had skied at Garmisch-Partenkirchen, Germany, and Stowe, Vermont. A native of Wisconsin, after military service and business school, he returned with a dream of revitalizing the stagnant economy of his hometown, where the fortunes of the logging industry had greatly declined. Wise says, "It seemed to me that recreational tourism was the way to go." In 1947, Wise decided to acquire a parcel of land at Cable, Wisconsin, which he planned to develop as an Alpine ski resort. He would call the resort Telemark, in honor of the Norwegian province where some people say skiing began. Never mind that he would be promoting skiing in an area only known for its summer recreational facilities, and that the highest hill on this land rose just 370 feet. The idea seemed so outlandish that the original owner of the parcel figured Wise was up to something. Hardly anybody in Wisconsin even knew what a ski resort was in those days. Once he convinced the wily farmer who owned the land that he hadn't discovered a rumored vein of silver, Wise was able to purchase the 120-acre plot, with its hillock, for just $750.

Despite its puny ski slope, Telemark was a good business venture. The cheap land made the initial investment low, and in 1947 skiing was not developed the way it is now. Back then, you couldn't hop on a jet in Minneapolis and land a few hours later near a Colorado ski resort. At first, his competition would be regional only. Over the next twenty-five years he built Telemark into one of the foremost skiing facilities of the Midwest. The farmer who once owned the hillside later became an employee and told Tony Wise, "I didn't sell you a silver mine, I sold you a gold mine."

Alpine skiing boomed during the 1960s, and that helped Telemark; but vacation travel by jet also boomed during the 1960s, and that didn't help. By 1970, midwestern skiers began to feel the strong lure of Rocky Mountain highs at Vail and Aspen. Undaunted, in 1972 Wise invested $6 million in a gigantic ski lodge at Telemark, which Billy Kidd, the Olympic downhill medalist, said was "bigger than the ski hill!" Designed by Herb Fritz, a disciple of Frank Lloyd Wright, the lodge won critical acclaim for its architecture. But how was Wise going to fill two hundred rooms?

Over the years Wise had picked up some street smarts, and the Harvard Business School probably didn't hurt either. He assessed his situation and commissioned a study on the feasibility of marketing a sport that was then relatively unknown in the United States, cross-country skiing. The undulating hills and forests around Cable, Wisconsin, were ideal for Nordic skiing, and the American popularity of that sport seemed to be growing. But was it possible to develop the demand for a first-class, cross-country ski facility?

The analysis revealed that only 30,000 pairs of cross-country skis had been sold that year, whereas 900,000 pairs of downhill skis had been sold. Still, upward trends in the popularity of cross-country ski equipment looked promising, so Wise sent Telemark's manager and assistant manager on a reconnaissance mission to Colorado, where some cross-country facilities already existed. Then Wise hired Sven Wiik, the cross-country skiing coach for the 1960 U.S. Olympic squad, to design trails. Wiik also recommended that Telemark stage a cross-country skiing event to promote the trails.

For years, Carl Hanson, a Swedish-American friend, had kept Wise informed of the many thousands of people who skied each year at the Vasaloppet in Mora, Sweden. On the advice of Wiik and Hanson, Wise announced a race. Since his own heritage and the theme of his lodge were Norwegian, Wise named the event after the Birkebeiner-Rennet. Initially, Wise had no premonition that participation in his own event, the American Birkebeiner, would eventually be comparable to participation in its Swedish and Norwegian counterparts. The first American Birkebeiner, on February 24, 1973, had only fifty-four participants, thirty-five who skied 50 kilometers and nineteen who skied a less demanding, short-distance event. (In later years, the smaller event was standardized at 29 kilometers and given the Swedish name Korteloppet, or short race.) Wise's Birkebeiner was low-key the first year. The greatest expenses in 1973 were for blueberry soup (which was a tradition of Scandinavian events), four Westclox timers, and crepe paper to tie around trees as course markers.

Many American cross-country skiing events predate the Birkebeiner, and even the name Birkebeiner itself had been used for a race sponsored by the Bemidji, Minnesota, chapter of the Sons of Norway. The first few years the United States Ski Association (USSA) was reluctant to even sanction the race, because the 55-kilometer distance seemed excessive and nonmembers were permitted to race. The former rationale appears strange, because by international standards the American Birkebeiner is not that long. The Grenader in Norway and the König Ludwig Lauf in West Germany are both 90 kilometers, and the Canadian Ski Marathon is a 120-kilometer event that requires two days.

Despite the USSA's initial refusal to sanction the "Birkie," the event was cleverly promoted and very consistent with the *Zeitgeist* of 1970s athletics. The spirit of mid-seventies sports favored endurance-length events and participation by large numbers of nonelite athletes. The USSA's apparent disdain for the "citizen" skier almost cost it an opportunity, but when that organization came on board, both the USSA and the Birkebeiner benefited. Even though the USSA demanded segregation of the elite athletes from the thundering herd of citizen skiers, the participation of champion-caliber skiers from Europe and America brought publicity and increased enrollment in the Birkebeiner.

As participation climbed, corporate sponsorship of the event fell into place, and the companies in turn used their public relations firms and considerable advertising leverage with national media to obtain coverage of the cross-country race. The publicity in turn made the event more popular. Popularity inspired still more publicity, and some people began to call the Boston Marathon "the Birkebeiner of running." Wise's event was a snowball rolling downhill; from 54 skiers in 1973, participation in the Birkebeiner and the shorter Korteloppet had steadily risen to 8,007 by 1984. Meanwhile, by that year U.S. cross-country ski purchases had risen to 600,000 pairs, a quantity approximately equal to the number of downhill ski purchases. Wise had called the correct shot when he bet on cross-country.

Wise also did clever things to promote his race. He founded the *Birch Scroll*, a magazine to publicize the race and solicit attendance at upcoming races. Unlike some long-distance events in skiing and other sports, the Birkebeiner has always supported participation by female athletes, and that further enhanced the event's appeal. Wise showed a flair for publicity and promotion, enhancing Birkebeiner hoopla with exhibition sprint races by the elite skiers, spaghetti feeds, pancake breakfasts, and training clinics. All entrants get to participate in a truly international "opening ceremony," whose pageantry is patterned after the Olympics. In the gala awards ceremony the last finisher is extolled and given the "bronzed broom award." Everybody gets a

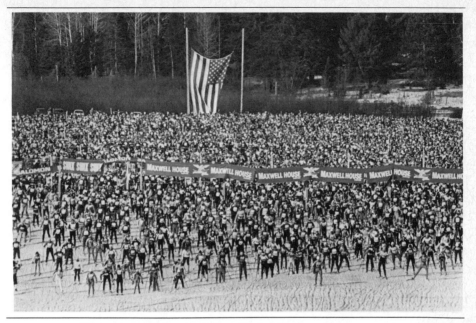

Wave start of the American Birkebeiner.
COURTESY OF AMERICAN BIRKEBEINER SKI FOUNDATION, INC.

finisher's medal. Wise even commissioned Englebert Hattenberger, an Austrian ice sculptor, to carve crowd-pleasing heroic frozen statues during the weekend of the event.

When the number of entries outgrew the ski trail, causing bottle-necks on the course and many collisions, Wise convinced the local government that the economic benefits of his race justified a public works project to build a new ski trail across public lands. In 1976, Sawyer County, Wisconsin, kicked in $20,000 and obtained $30,000 in federal matching funds to cut a forest trail wide enough to accommodate fifteen skiers across. Telemark Resort had to pay for a 5-kilometer section of trail entering neighboring Bayfield County, which declined to contribute to the project but allowed an easement for the trail.

Enrollment continued to climb, again causing gridlock on the ski trail by 1978. In 1979, this time with the participation of Bayfield County as well as Sawyer County and the federal government, an additional $94,000 was spent to widen the trail to permit thirty skiers abreast.

Early in the history of the race, Wise established contacts with the Norwegian Birkebeiner. The race has fostered ties between people in Wisconsin and Norway. Cultural exchanges, such as free trips to the Norwegian event by the winner of the Birkie's citizen race, led eventually to hundreds of Norwegians flying to Wise's event on special air tours. Exploiting the Norwegian connection was smart politics in the Birkie's Wisconsin venue. Many of the potential entrants were Scandinavian-Americans who are fiercely proud of their roots.

Wise was instrumental in creating the Worldloppet, a series of ten ski races in ten different countries.* The American Birkebeiner is the United States race, and the series includes races in Finland, Norway, Sweden, Italy, Austria, Switzerland, West Germany, France, and Canada. Citizen skiers can obtain Worldloppet Master Diplomas by purchasing Worldloppet Passports for $25 and then getting them stamped for completing each of the ten races at least once during their skiing careers. As of 1985, 1,753 citizen skiers had joined Worldloppet and 173 had completed all ten races. Elite skiers also compete for the annual Worldloppet Cup prize. The cup goes to the skier with the most points in six of that winter's races. The six events must include loppets in North America, Scandinavia, and middle Europe.

It has been proposed that a race in the Soviet Union, the Murmansk Ski Marathon, become the eleventh race in the Worldloppet. The Russian race is a highlight of a civic celebration at the end of the bitter winter in Murmansk. That city is the largest ice-free port north of the Arctic Circle. The Russians call their celebration "the Festival of the Peoples of the North." It includes reindeer-sled racing as well as the 58-kilometer ski marathon, which attracts seven thousand "comrade" skiers. For the moment it appears that poor East-West relations will prevent the Russians from joining this international sports federation. The Europeans are strongly opposed to Soviet inclusion, although U.S. delegates do not object to the Russians joining Worldloppet.

Since 1979, the American Birkebeiner has also been part of a strictly American cross-country ski series called the Great American Ski Chase, which encompasses eight races in New England, Colorado, the Midwest, and Montana. All of those events are 50 kilometers or longer. Endurance skiing has clearly blossomed in America.

Success of the Birkie is not entirely attributable to Tony Wise and his ski lodge. Long-distance skiing was an idea whose time had come. Other endurance sports were experiencing similar growth, and in many places some of those sports—such as running and cycling—are difficult to do during the winter. Cross-country skiing is an ideal off-season activity for cyclists and runners. The silver medal that Bill Koch won at the 1976 Innsbruck Winter Olympics also inspired many Americans to take up cross-country skiing. No American before Koch had ever won an Olympic medal for Nordic racing.

---

*When first founded in 1978, the Worldloppet included only nine events. In 1980, the Worldloppet committee added a race in France, the 76-kilometer (47.2-mile) Transjurassienne.

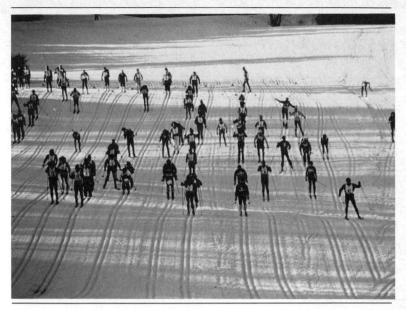

A cross-country event in France.   PHOTO BY SYLVIE CHAPPAZ

Even technology was on Wise's side; fiberglass had the same impact on skiing as that material had on rowing and pole vaulting. Some of the new fiberglass Nordic skis permit skiing without waxing the bottoms. (Although best results are still achieved by waxing, the arcane mysteries of deciding which wax to use for each type of snow had previously intimidated some novices.) Similarly, fiberglass ski poles are much stronger, more flexible, and easier to handle than their bamboo predecessors.

Of course, the burgeoning participation in cross-country skiing may be a mixed blessing. According to surveys by skiing magazines, the vast majority of Nordic skiers rate a scenic ski course as the most important attraction of an event. It's hard to enjoy the scenery when you are in a traffic jam on skis. Some long-time Nordic skiers resent the commercial exploitation and mass marketing of what had been a solitary, contemplative sport for them. Nonetheless, anybody who dislikes mass participation events is free to avoid them, and it still is possible for Nordic skiers to find lonely wilderness trails to ski by themselves. Also, some events, such as the 40-kilometer Steamboat Stampede in Steamboat Springs, Colorado, are still well-kept secrets, attracting no more than a hundred participants.* What is more, the

*You can obtain information about cross-country skiing events by contacting the United States Ski Association, 1750 East Boulder Street, Colorado Springs, CO 80909. *Cross Country Skier* is a publication with valuable information on the sport. Subscription inquiries for that bimonthly magazine should be addressed to Rodale Press, 33 East Minor Street, Emmaus, PA 18049.

heavily attended long-distance events give skiers that much more incentive to put in training time by themselves or in a small group on isolated trails. The crowded events then become personal endurance tests, and the mass constituency gives manufacturers the financial incentive to keep improving equipment.

The future for endurance skiing generally seems very bright. There will be more events, more developed and supported ski trails, more skiers and better equipment.

Unfortunately, the future for both Tony Wise and his American Birkebeiner are not as certain. Developing the event and his ski resort, Wise went way out on a limb financially. Wise does things first-class, and that takes money. During the years of high interest rates in the 1970s and early 1980s, he borrowed heavily. Although the event grew steadily, recession and several winters with poor snow hurt the resort's business. Wise has lost the Telemark Lodge, and at least for the moment the Birkebeiner too, in bankruptcy proceedings. The event continues, although Wise has been outspoken in his bitter criticism of the committee that now puts it on. He calls them "a Quisling rump group," an epithet that will be readily understood by Norwegian-Americans in Hayward, Wisconsin.

For their part, the Birkebeiner Foundation and the present operators of Telemark point with pride to the fact that they are perpetuating Wise's creation, an event that is important to the local economy and the continued growth of endurance skiing. Confusion over the controversy has reduced Birkebeiner registration, but the event will probably endure.

As for Wise, he is down, but don't count him out. He still is an endurance-event promoter extraordinaire. He is the motivating force behind American Classic Competitions, a corporation that promotes a multisport endurance series that includes the Tour de Raddison, a 350-kilometer bike race; the Muskelunge Swim, a 6-kilometer event; the Log-Driver Half Marathon; and the 42-kilometer Leif Erikson Roller Ski Race (for off-season skiers who want to do roadwork). Although Wise doesn't own the Birkebeiner anymore, scores in that event round out the cumulative point total for series participants. Those who complete all five races in one year have a shot at winning the American Classic Championship. The events of the series add up to about 294 miles.

To compete with his old Worldloppet, Wise is now trying to start a Cosmosloppet, including countries not now in the Worldloppet, such as Iceland, Spain, New Zealand, Japan, and the Eastern-bloc nations.

Wise also holds the Lumberjack World Championships, a nationally televised event that perpetuates the macho skills of woodcutters, which largely have been mechanized out of existence. The championship includes events such as log rolling, log splitting, pole climbing, and buck sawing. Wise claims that some of the lumberjacks saw so fast and hard that they bleed from their noses.

Recently *Ultrasport* magazine gave Wise an award for his skill as a sports impresario. *Ultrasport* placed his name alongside those of Mike Aisner, the promoter of the Coors Classic bicycle race; Fred Lebow, of New York City Marathon fame; Valerie Silk, the highly regarded director of the Ironman Triathlon; and Bob Eiger, ABC Sports' director of program planning. Even if he doesn't make a comeback, Wise's name will always be in good company.

ICE IS NICE

Ice skating is to Holland as skiing is to Scandinavia. It is a national passion. From 1909 until 1963 the Dutch held an annual 200-kilometer (120-mile) speed-skating race called the Elfstedentocht, which means Eleven Cities Tour. The race existed informally as far back as 1763. Since 1963, the ice on the canals has not been reliable for skating, and large numbers of Dutch have flown wherever necessary to hold their endurance contest—Norway, Finland, the United States, and Canada.

Weather conditions for the race have varied from bad to awful. Two contestants died of exposure and only 58 of the 10,227 starters finished the 1963 race. The winner of the 1929 race lost his big toe to frostbite, but winners of the Elfstedentocht are national heroes, so he was able to prevail upon his family to preserve the toe in a jar for fifty years after the race.

The Dutch skating classic came to the United States in 1983, when it was staged on Lake Memphremagog, a beautiful body of water sandwiched between Canada on the north and the fading Vermont resort town of Newport on the south. That race was won by Jan Roelof Kruithof, a forty-seven-year-old architect who has won the Eleven Cities Tour many times before.

Since its moment in the limelight of international sports, Newport has been the site of other endurance skating contests. When ice conditions permit, the Newport Winterfest now includes an annual ice-skating marathon, whose distance varies according to weather and ice conditions. (In 1985 it was 40 kilometers.)

Newport has joined with the Canadian cities of Montreal, Ottawa, and Quebec to form the Canadian American Marathon Skating Association (CAMSA). CAMSA promotes and sanctions long-distance skating events in the two countries.

KEEP THE CRANKS TURNING

Bicycling is an unusual endurance sport in that most people learn to ride a bicycle, yet relatively few people enter bicycle races. Possibly the skill and fancy equipment required and the physical risks of competing at close quarters have prevented many amateur athletes from racing bicycles. Hence, competitive cycling hasn't quite developed the mass constituency that exists for running events and cross-country ski races. Typically, cyclists use their bicycles for transportation, commuting, recreation, long-distance touring, or exercise. Bicycling is reputed to be the number-two participation sport. But because the goal of preparing for an event is absent, many cyclists don't train with the same religious regularity as do runners, swimmers, and other endurance athletes.

Lately there are indications that public participation in bicycle racing is on the rise. A few "citizen" races and mass tours, which some riders treat as races, have sprung up. An example is the Tecate-Ensenada Bike Race, a 72-mile cycling carnival in Mexico's Baja, which begins in the border town of Tecate, near San Diego, California. When David Manwaring founded the event in 1970, he was one of nine riders who participated. Since then his annual race has grown to include an estimated twelve thousand riders, from virtually all walks of life. Participation fluctuates slightly from year to year, as tourism is affected by such factors as peso devaluation and threats of violence against gringos. The riders range from world-class cyclists, who finish in about three hours, to "completers," who require as many as twelve hours (and afterward may hang up their bikes for good).

The Tecate-Ensenada course includes some challenging hills, bumpy mountain roads, and a fairly consistent head wind, caused by an onshore breeze from the nearby Pacific Ocean. The raucous spectators, who greatly outnumber participants, and the antics of some riders manage to turn the endurance event into a party. A few Tecate-Ensenada cyclists ride in costumes, and bicycles vary from sleek, imported racing machines to beach bombers and turn-of-the-century, high-wheeled "ordinaries." So far, the Mexicans tolerate the event because of its economic benefits. Still, the clash of cultures and values sometimes is embarrassing. One can only hope that the endurance required by the ride will tone down the ugly-American behavior without suppressing the festive ambience.

The rapidly growing sport of triathlon has given many athletes a taste of bicycling, and that has helped broaden the support base for competitive cycling. Yet bike racing still remains largely a spectator sport. In Europe the popularity of professional bike racing is eclipsed only by that of soccer. In the United States, bicycling is a relatively minor spectator sport, although it had a greater following than baseball in the early years of this century. Amateur participation and the success of American cyclists at the 1984 Olympics have partly resurrected the earlier crowd appeal. Television coverage and other media attention to two events—the Tour de France and the Coors Classic—have also helped win fans for American cycling.

Both the Tour de France and the Coors Classic are stage races. A stage race is a bicycle road event in which the cyclists cover a long distance in a series of separate races during a period of a few days or several weeks. The stages might include criteriums, or repeated laps around a relatively short loop; time trials, in which each cyclist embarks separately and rides against the clock; as well as the straightforward long-distance road-race stages.

Vive Les Cyclistes!

The Tour de France has a long and illustrious history, but it was created by and for the media. In 1903, Henri Desgrange's sporting newspaper *L'Auto* was locked in a no-holds-barred circulation war with *Le Velo*, the sponsor of two popular nonstop, endurance bike races—the 700-mile Paris-Brest-Paris and the 400-mile Bordeaux-Paris. Desgrange, who had been a champion cyclist before he became a publisher, created a stage race to upstage his competitor. He offered twenty thousand francs in prize money—an award that would be worth $44,500 at 1985 prices—and concocted a month-long cycling extravaganza. His Tour de France Cycliste was a 1,500-mile circuit of France: Paris-Lyon-Marseille-Toulouse-Bordeaux-Nantes-Paris. (Way ahead of his time, the ex-competitor also used the event to campaign for fitness.)

Desgrange's gambit worked: the tour was a smashing success. It drew a gigantic crowd wherever it went, and the appetite for his newspaper's official coverage was so great that circulation doubled. (*L'Auto* still publishes and promotes the Tour under its modern name, *L'Équipe*, or "team" in English.)

From this very auspicious beginning, the Tour has grown still more in distance, public interest, financial importance, and prestige. The longest Tour de France was a 5,757-kilometer (3,569-mile) race contested over twenty-nine days in 1926, but now the Tour lasts twenty-three days and usually covers about 3,900 kilometers (2,400 miles). Still, that is 900 miles longer than the first Tour. Except during the two world wars, the Tour has been staged each July since 1903. (Traditionally, July 14, Bastille Day, is a day off from the Tour.)

Tour winners share prizes in excess of $300,000, but a winner usually gives all or most of his money to his nine teammates, including the "domestiques," who might have burned themselves out providing wind blockage to help him catch a breakaway, may have given him a wheel when he flatted, or might have sacrificed their own race by relinquishing a bicycle when he crashed. The stars of the Tour get their financial rewards in generous appearance money for racing in numerous 100-kilometer exhibition criteriums during the month following the Tour. Winning at the Tour also enables riders to renew their contracts with automobile, ice cream, wine, and other manufacturers who sponsor the teams. Greg LeMond, whose second-place finish in 1985 made him the most successful American Tour rider ever, has a $1.2 million, four-year contract with his sponsor, La Vie Claire.

La Vie Claire is a chain of French health food stores owned by Bernard Tapie, a flamboyant entrepreneur who specializes in acquiring and revitalizing ailing companies. He has helped promote that company by sponsoring the most successful professional cycling team in the world.

LeMond's contract makes him the highest-paid cyclist in history. The team also includes Bernard Hinault, one of the best professional riders of this century.

In 1919, the Tour began allowing the rider with the lowest cumulative time for previous stages to wear a yellow jersey *(le maillot jaune)*. Winning the yellow jersey can be a great honor for a rider who may not go on to win the race, because he is less skilled in some later phase of the Tour (such as hill climbing). It is possible to win all but the last stage and still lose the overall honors to some other rider who went much faster than you on that final stage. Winning the yellow jersey twelve days in a row, Vincent Barteau of the Renault team wore it for more stages of the 1984 Tour than any other rider, but it was his teammate Laurent Fignon who won that year's Tour de France. Fignon didn't wear *le maillot jaune* until the eighteenth stage of the twenty-three-stage event. Indeed, it is possible to win by having the lowest final total even though you never wore the yellow jersey. As Yogi Berra said, "It ain't over till it's over."

Following a practice instituted in the 1930s, the coveted white jersey with red polka dots is designated to honor the King of the Mountains, the best hill climber.

The present system, whereby most teams are sponsored by manufacturers, was instituted in 1962, when the national teams were disallowed. It was unrealistic to ask professional cyclists to abandon alliances and financial obligations to their normal multinational teams in order to represent an ad-hoc patriotic team. Since that step, the race promoters have experimented with allowing national teams, and national amateur teams are now permitted.

In 1984 the Tour de France broke an eighty-one-year tradition

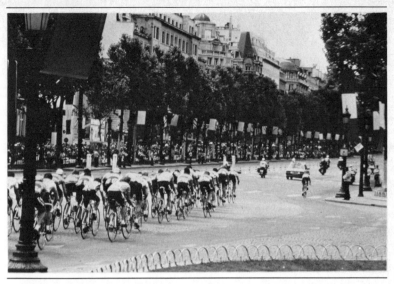

The Tour de France.   COURTESY OF ALL-SPORT/VANDYSTADT

and permitted women to race. Five nations, the United States, Canada, Holland, France, and Great Britain sent amateur teams.* (Since very little prize money exists for women's cycling events, there are virtually no female professionals, only amateurs.) Mary Ann Martin (USA) won the event.

Le Tour de France Féminin was completely separated from the men's race, permitting individual recognition for the women, who generally are slower road racers than men. Unfortunately, the women's stages also were only about half the length of the men's stages. There is nothing inherently wrong with a race half as long as the men's Tour, but this decision appears to be inspired by the erroneous belief that women are not suited for endurance athletics. Perhaps Tour director Félix Lévitan thought that the women's Tour would not be successful if some women couldn't finish a longer course. The small number of contestants would have made any failures conspicuous. However, many men fail to finish the Tour, and that only *adds* to the drama.

Some riders, such as Canada's Jacqueline Shaw, who is an ultradistance specialist, hoped that the Tour Féminin would be lengthened, but instead the women's course was shortened a bit more for the 1985 race. For the moment it appears the women's event will be a middle-distance stage race.

Over the years, the Tour de France has continually evolved, but one characteristic has remained constant: during the Tour, nothing else in France matters very much. An estimated 15 to 20 million Europeans are on the sidelines of the Tour for at least one stage. Many

*France was represented by two teams, making six in all.

millions more tune in to the six or seven hours of live, daily television coverage. Gossip about the Tour and its riders fills the front pages of French newspapers. A throng mobs the Champs Élysées for the traditional finish of the Tour. (The Tour is the only event for which that avenue is officially closed). A huge entourage, including support personnel for the ten-member teams, journalists, representatives of team sponsors, and itinerant fans, follows the entire Tour. A commercial caravan entertaining the masses with song and dance, selling merchandise, advertising products, and passing out samples precedes each stage.

Civic pride and the financial benefits to businesses in Tour cities are so great that the towns of France battle fiercely to be included. In America, athletic event promoters often must reimburse municipalities for such services as police protection, but in France it works the other way around. Cities pay dearly for the privilege of being a stage stop on the Tour.

The riders, who endure a grueling twenty-three-day schedule of races averaging more than 100 miles, are the ones responsible for making the Tour the Super Bowl of France. As Americans remember Ty Cobb, the French remember Eugene Cristophe, whose fans called him Cri-Cri. Cristophe broke his bicycle's fork in the 1913 and 1919 Tours, but on both occasions repaired it himself at blacksmith shops and reentered the race. In 1919 he thought his heroic response to the calamity had been awarded by a Tour victory, but later he was penalized ten minutes (and thus lost the race) because a young boy had operated the bellows at the smith's forge. Nowadays you can receive a whole new bicycle in the field, but in those days the rules proscribed any mechanical assistance.

Fausto Coppi and Louison Bobet were beloved Tour champions because their riding had "heart." An advocate of scientific training, Coppi won two Tours in the years after World War II, as well as five Giro d'Italias. (The Giro, Italy's Tour, was founded in 1909.) In the 1955 Tour, Bobet defied doctors' orders by riding in a swelteringly hot hill-climbing stage over Mont Ventoux, despite excruciating saddle sores. The riders attacked each other fiercely that day, mindless of the oppressive heat. Before the stage was over one opponent, Jean Mallejac, was in a coma, and another, Ferdi Kubler, finished the race nearly unconscious. But Bobet won the Mont Ventoux stage and went on to win the Tour. In all, Bobet won three Tours.

Other Tour champions had only the grudging respect of the fans. In 1964, when he won his fifth Tour—a feat that so far has been replicated by only Eddy Merckx and Bernard Hinault—Jacques Anquetil actually was jeered by the French fans, because they believed he did no more than was necessary to win the overall victory. Many fans also disliked Bernard Hinault, who dominated the Tour for seven years, winning it four times between 1978 and 1982 and again taking top honors in 1985. His riding is perceived as calculating and lacking in panache because he doesn't pursue flashy victories in difficult stages such as those in the mountains. Yet he holds the record for the fastest average speed in a Tour de France, 23.5 miles per hour in 1981. Those fans want blood!

In the 1985 Tour, he gave them blood. That year he chalked up his fifth victory, despite a handlebar tangle with Australian rider Phil Anderson as they were sprinting to the finish of a stage in St. Étienne. Hinault's face bounced several times on the pavement, and he broke his nose in two places. But he got up, finished the stage, rode a mountain stage in the Pyrenees the next day, and went on to win the Tour. He has shown his courage, if not his panache, and probably will back off in future Tours to allow his La Vie Claire teammate, the American Greg LeMond, to capture some of the glory.

A fellow cyclist nicknamed Hinault *le blaireau*, the badger. The cycling press has made that epithet stick, because the badger is a strong animal that can be very nasty when cornered. Hinault could win virtually any stage of the tour, including the mountain stages, but he is unexcelled as a time trialist. Hence, he sometimes strategically allows other riders to take victories, making up the deficit in the time trials. Hinault believes that consistently good performances in each of the Tour's diverse stages is the key to victory, and in 1983 sagely told *The New York Times Magazine* interviewer Samuel Abt, "I race to last, not to finish broken." Spoken like a true endurance athlete.

To European fans Belgian rider Eddy Merckx is the Babe Ruth of cycling. "The cannibal," as they call him, was renowned for his ferocious competitiveness, and he is one of the three riders who has won the Tour five times. Merckx was victorious in the Tour from 1969 through 1972 and again in 1974. He has been known to gratuitously increase his margin of victory on stages he already had in the bag, thereby jeopardizing his performance on subsequent days. Merckx earned permanent adulation for the courage he showed in the 1975 Tour. A fanatical spectator assaulted him during one stage of that Tour, but Merckx persevered and finished the Tour in the number-two position in spite of liver injuries and a broken jaw.

Later Merckx again showed tolerance for pain. On October 25, 1972, he went to Mexico City to pursue one of the most coveted and difficult records in cycling, "the Hour." The air in Mexico City, whose elevation is 7,414 feet, is 20 percent less dense than that at sea level, and on balance that is an advantage for setting cycling records. The lower air resistance more than compensates for the athlete's greater difficulty getting enough air to breathe. But Merckx pushed himself excruciatingly close to his physical limits. Circling an oval velodrome, he cycled 49.714 kilometers (30 miles and 3,770 yards), setting a record that stood until 1984. When he was done he could not support his own weight, and he exclaimed that the effort was so painful that he would never attempt "the Hour" again, even though he was tantalizingly close to the elusive 50-kilometer barrier.

On January 23, 1984, Italy's Francesco Moser broke the 50-kilometer barrier. Moser's new world record of 51.151 kilometers (31 miles and 1,381 yards) was controversial because he used disk wheels. Conventional spoked wheels churn up the air the way an eggbeater whips cream. At 30 miles per hour, aerodynamic factors constitute at least 90 percent of the total forces retarding a bicycle's forward motion. Disk wheels provide a substantial advantage, but is it a "legal" advantage? Since the 1930s, the organization that governs international cycling, the Union Cycliste International (UCI), has banned streamlined bicycles because they provide an unfair competitive advantage. The UCI ruled in favor of Moser's disk wheels, however, and recognized the new record. Still, Merckx's record stood unchallenged for almost a dozen years, and up to this writing nobody has bettered it on a bicycle with standard spoked wheels.

Herb Tea, Beer, and Bicycles in the Rockies

Unlike the situation in Europe, America's professional bicycle racing had fallen victim to automobile mania and baseball's popularity by the 1930s. Motorpaced events—in which cyclists raced around banked oval tracks in the slipstreams of motorcycles—survived in America up to the 1920s. In Europe motorpacing is still popular. America's six-day bike races flourished throughout the 1920s. In the twenties, the renown of six-day biker Alf Goullet—an Australian-American now ninety-four years old—rivaled that of his contemporaries, Jack Dempsey and Babe Ruth, but by 1940 his sport succumbed to what Goullet calls a "ham and eggs" style of promotion. In Europe six-day bike racing continues. Only amateur cycling survives intact in America, and until the recent growth of endurance sport, cycling has taken a back seat to many other American sports. Hence, it is not surprising that America's Coors Classic has a much shorter history and a much less fanatical following than the Tour de France.

In 1975, Mo Siegal was a twenty-five-year-old hip capitalist, whose Boulder, Colorado, business, the Celestial Seasonings Herb Tea Company, was stocking the shelves of health food stores with its Red Zinger tea. The wave of idealism, pacifism, and love that swept across America in the 1960s had largely receded by 1975, but little tidal pools of huru-guru enlightenment linger to this day in places like Colorado. Mo Siegal no doubt saw some cosmic connection between mind-expanding bicycle races in the mountains and his herbal teas. Hence, Celestial Seasonings created a race, the Red Zinger Bicycle Classic.

The race has flourished, as has Siegal's company, which he recently unloaded for an undisclosed six-figure sum. Siegal's event now carries the name of a stronger beverage than tea. Since 1980 the Adolph Coors Brewery has sponsored the race.

The Coors Bicycle Classic is an amateur stage race for men and women; it has attracted Olympic-caliber riders such as America's Alexi Grewal and Connie Carpenter, and France's Jeannie Longo. John Howard, who dominated American amateur cycling in the 1970s, won the event twice when it was still the Red Zinger. The American wun-derkind Greg LeMond, who has taken European professional cycling by storm, also has been a winner.

In 1985, the Coors Classic took a step toward the national scope that characterizes the Tour de France. Whereas all previous Coors Classics had been confined to Colorado, the 1985 race started in San Francisco and finished in Colorado.

The Citizen Cyclist

From an endurance-athletics point of view, the Coors Classic and Tour de France can be criticized because they are strictly elite races. Hence, for most of us, they are only spectator events. Lately, a new form of endurance bicycle racing has developed, and it shows promise of lead-ing to citizen racing. That new form is nonstop cross-American racing.

John Marino has been called the father of transcontinental bike racing. In his youth, Marino would never have predicted his future role in endurance sport. He was an athlete all right, but his main sport was baseball. From his junior high school days, his greatest ambition was to play major-league baseball. (His position was catcher.) He was an okay batter, but most important, Marino had a good throwing arm and could run from home plate to first base in about 3.5 seconds. John explains that coaching can improve your batting, but you either have a good arm or you don't, and there's very little that a team can do about your natural potential for speed.

The Dodgers tried to draft him during his freshman year at a junior college near Los Angeles. Unfortunately, they offered him a very small bonus as an incentive to sign. It's a general rule in profes-sional sports that the effort a team expends on bringing a rookie along is proportional to the initial investment. Marino rejected their offer, figuring he was only nineteen years old and could more advantageously

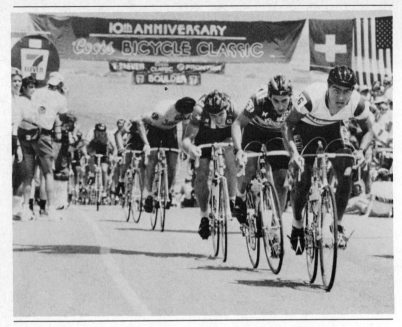

The mountainous Morgul-Bismarck stage of the Coors Classic is infamous for its finish atop the "wall." Here Mexican Raul Acala is chased up the "wall" by 1984 winner, Doug Shapiro.

PHOTO BY JULIAN BAUM, COURTESY OF COORS BICYCLE CLASSIC

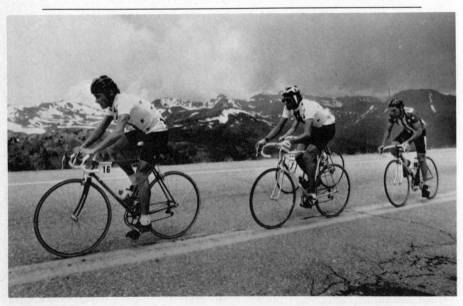

At the 1984 Coors Classic, Olympic gold medalist Alexi Grewal and Doug Shapiro, the eventual race winner, chase Jeff Pierce across 12,000-foot Loveland Pass.

PHOTO BY MICHAEL CHRITTON, COURTESY OF COORS BICYCLE CLASSIC

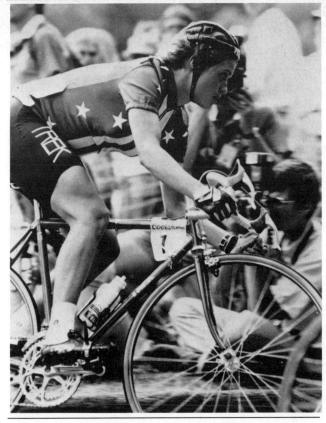

Rebecca Twigg, Olympic silver medalist and winner of the 1983 Coors Classic.

PHOTO BY JULIAN BAUM, COURTESY OF COORS BICYCLE CLASSIC

join the team later if he continued to develop. He played semipro ball with the Dodgers' winter league and kept his options open to pursue other sports. He had one eye cast toward football.

Partly because he wanted to beef up for football, Marino had begun to pump iron. He worked out as a power lifter, and was eventually able to lift several hundred pounds. Although his training was adequate for most power lifting, Marino understates the matter when he says, "Sometimes I bite off more than I can chew." On one occasion he was dead lifting 525 pounds, when something went terribly wrong. Other people at the weight room heard a sharp, loud snap from Marino's lower back, and the next thing he knew the barbell had bounced off the gym floor and he was numbly sitting with his legs shaking. He got up and tried to walk around, but suddenly his back was in excruciating pain. The doctor diagnosed Marino's injury as a compression fracture of the last lumbar vertebra and the sacrum and told him that he was finished with competitive sports. That was the last thing John wanted to hear.

Marino slowly recuperated and kept trying to return to baseball. Two years after the injury, it seemed as though he might prove the doctor wrong. He went to spring training in Phoenix, Arizona, to try out for the Oakland club. He did his best, but back pain returned during batting practice and anytime he attempted to run farther than half a mile. He was cut from the squad.

Marino's dream of glory on the baseball diamond was at an end. He says, "I drove back to Los Angeles, hung my mitt up, and decided to go to Europe for as long as I wanted to stay." He bought a one-way steamship ticket and committed himself to partying in Europe. He traveled from one European tourist attraction to another for about a year and a half, working when necessary. He drank a lot of beer, completely dropped all athletic training, and gained about 30 pounds.

Then, just for the novelty, he chose the bicycle as a means of travel from Frankfurt to Athens. He recalls, "When I took up bicycling it was not as a sport, but as a means of transportation; I wasn't looking at bicycling as a way to get in shape." But on that tour, Marino discovered that riding didn't adversely affect his back injury and that cycling long distances definitely could get him into good physical condition.

Nonetheless, when he completed that long ride in Europe, Marino resumed his sedentary habits. He still had his back problems too. On one frightening occasion, after he returned to America, he experienced back spasms severe enough to prevent him from walking. A girl friend talked him into seeing a chiropractor, who scolded him for being overweight and out of shape. The chiropractor claimed that the twenty-five-year-old ex-jock's poor physical condition was the reason why he had not recovered from the injury. As a remedy to the problem, the chiropractor recommended a vegetarian diet and exercise. Initially Marino was skeptical. But since mainstream therapies had failed, he resolved to follow the chiropractor's advice. Marino believes that losing weight, resuming exercise, and frequently obtaining deep muscle massage greatly improved his back condition.

At about this point in his life, Marino also began to attend various motivational courses and lectures. In particular he says he was influenced by one guru's "auto-generational acquisition theory." Partly because Marino was unhappy and disillusioned with his present occupation—substitute teaching—the motivational training convinced him that he should seek a world record in athletics. He had recently tried running as a sport, but it aggravated his old lower back injury. Almost as one might pick a gift from a catalog, Marino browsed through

The Guinness Book of Records until Paul Cornish's thirteen-day, five-hour, and twenty-minute record for bicycling across America caught his eye. Marino quit his job and began training in earnest.

In 1978, and again in 1980, Marino set new records for bicycling across the country (thirteen days, one hour, and twenty minutes; and twelve days, three hours, forty-one minutes). On these rides he was accompanied by a support team in a motor home, but he raced against no other riders. Although his competition was only the clock, his determination was so impressive that McGraw-Hill produced *Psychling*, a prize-winning motivational film about the 1980 ride.

When Lon Haldeman, a bike-shop mechanic from Harvard, Illinois, took more than a day off Marino's record the next year, Marino decided to act on an earlier idea. Since Haldeman was competing against him anyway, why not start a head-to-head race. Marino had gone into debt to finance his 1978 ride and had broken even because of a bicycle company's sponsorship in 1980. But the publicity of a real race might attract some prize money. Then he might be able to make a living doing his transcontinental rides.

Hence, in 1982 John Marino, Michael Shermer, Lon Haldeman, and John Howard decided to promote and race in a cross-American competition that they would call the Great American Bike Race (GABR). Bob Eiger, the producer of ABC's "Wide World of Sports," viewed Marino's motivational film, saw the potential for a show, and decided to cover the first transcontinental race. Lon Haldeman won the event, setting a new record of nine days, twenty hours, and two minutes, and ABC won an Emmy award for their show.

The new event was a hit, and three of the riders—Shermer, Marino, and Haldeman—wanted to repeat it the following year. But a dispute with an agent who had helped promote the GABR led the athletes to rename the 1983 event the Race Across AMerica (RAAM).

Competition often inspires performance improvements, and the RAAM has radically decreased the time it takes for a bicyclist to cross America. In 1984 Pete Penseyres, a nuclear engineer for whom cycling was merely a hobby, lowered the record almost another seven hours, to nine days, thirteen hours, thirteen minutes. Jonathan Boyer, the first American to ever race in the Tour de France, beat twenty-six other riders in the 1985 race with an amazing time of nine days, two hours, and six minutes. Boyer's victory was another quantum leap; he lowered Penseyres's record by nearly half a day.

How much faster can America be crossed by bicycle? The duration of the trip has been decreased by about four days between 1978 and 1985. As it stands, the riders hardly sleep at all during the RAAM. But Michael Shermer predicts that the nine-day barrier will be broken

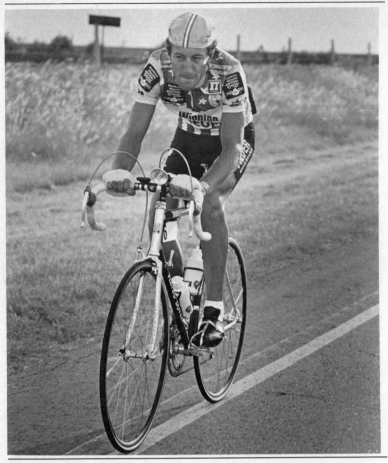

Jonathan Boyer, the first American permitted to race in the Tour de France, on his way to setting a transcontinental record and winning the 1985 Race Across AMerica.   PHOTO BY DAVE NELSON

in future RAAMs. Motorists often take longer than that to cross America.

Most people will never compete in the RAAM. But Shermer points out, "The average bike tourist can relate more to a RAAM rider than he can a Tour de France rider, because the RAAM is something he can do himself. He can envision himself out there on the highway crossing the country." The RAAM is likely to encourage citizen bike racing. True to its name, the RAAM's 700-mile qualifying race, the John Marino Open, is "open" to all entrants. The widely publicized and nationally televised RAAM has inspired other endurance races open to the general public, such as the 500-mile Spenco 500 in Texas. Of course 700-mile and 500-mile races are still a bit extreme for the average bicycle tourist, but during the past few years attendance at bike races longer than 100 miles has often exceeded one thousand riders. Shermer predicts, "The century and double-century rides will become the 10-k's of cycling."

Human-Powered Vehicles

Chester Kyle was an amateur master's-class bike racer and professor of mechanical engineering at California State University, Long Beach, when in 1973 he rediscovered some facts about bicycle aerodynamics that may revolutionize cycling. From 1933 to 1939, François Faure, a competitive track rider of only modest ability, broke virtually every existing cycling record. For instance, Faure rode 31.4 miles in one hour. How was it possible for a second-rank rider to rewrite the record books?

The answer is aerodynamics. Designed by M. Mochet, Faure's bicycle, the Vélocar, was a streamlined, supine recumbent. That is, the Vélocar was a low-slung bicycle on which the rider reclined—back downward—and pedaled with a push-pull motion. On the Vélocar, the air's resistance to Faure's motion was reduced by two factors: his recumbent position gave him a much smaller frontal profile than he would have on a conventional bicycle, and the fairings made the air flow around him smoothly rather than turbulently, as it would around an unfaired cyclist. As noted earlier, at racing speeds air resistance accounts for more than 90 percent of the retarding force that a bicyclist must overcome to make forward progress. On his aerodynamic bicycle, Faure had a substantial—some would say unfair—advantage over riders of regular bicycles. Of course, other cyclists could have imitated his bicycle, and their greater skill and strength would have set new records. Instead, bureaucrats took them away. In 1936, functionaries of the Union Cycliste International—the same organization that recently permitted Francesco Moser to use aerodynamic disk wheels—disallowed Faure's records and banned streamlined bicycles from future competition. Because of the rule change, bicycle streamlining was abandoned for almost four decades to follow.

By 1973, when Professor Kyle was doing mechanical engineering research on tire friction, Mochet's work and Faure's discredited records had been virtually forgotten. Since he was an amateur cyclist, Kyle used bicycles for his tire research, but air resistance was making it impossible to get the measurements he desired. He decided to streamline a bicycle and discovered serendipitously that doing so made the bicycle much more efficient. When he calculated some of the aerodynamic forces involved, he realized how much more powerful air resistance was than rolling resistance. He changed the focus of his research and began to build streamlined bikes.

The rest is history. Within a year Kyle had built a streamlined bicycle that Olympic cyclist Ron Skarin used to set a world record of 43.02 miles per hour for a 200-meter sprint at the Los Alamitos Naval Air Station. When Kyle sought recognition for Skarin's record, he came up against the UCI's stern admonition, and it was then that he learned of Mochet's previous streamlining efforts. Consistent with their earlier ruling, the UCI was unwilling to establish a special category for aerodynamic bicycles. About this time he also learned that other researchers—such as Los Angeles aeronautical engineer Jack Lambie—were also interested in streamlined bicycles. With Lambie and others, Kyle formed the International Human-Powered Vehicle Association (IHPVA)* as an organization to recognize records by bicycles whose design was unrestricted. As long as a vehicle was powered by human effort the IHPVA would recognize the records it set, regardless of the measures taken to cut down air resistance.

Staging the IHPVA speed championships over the next few years led to remarkable performances by human-powered vehicles (HPV's), with radically innovative aerodynamic designs. Some of the HPV's appeared to be the comic work of mad scientists. But nobody was laughing in 1980, when one vehicle, the Vector Tandem—a completely enclosed, sleek tricycle with two riders—set a record of 62.92 miles per hour for a 200-meter sprint. (Consider for comparison the 43.45-mile-per-hour record on conventional bikes, set by the Soviet cyclist Sergei Kopylov in 1982.)

Yet, 200-meter sprints hardly demonstrate anything about practical transportation, and the IHPVA is dominated by engineers interested in producing useful vehicles. The Vector Tandem's endurance qualities had to be tested if its usefulness was to be established.

A consistent problem for human-powered vehicles is ventilation. A working cyclist produces a lot of heat, and completely enclosed vehicles don't allow that heat to escape. On a sunny day there also is a greenhouse effect, as the sunlight penetrates the vehicle's windshield and the heat is trapped within. The riders of HPV's could cook on any but the shortest rides. Human-powered vehicles are designed with skirts that sweep the pavement to keep ground-turbulence effects from increasing aerodynamic drag. Unfortunately, the skirts further compromise ventilation because they purposely reduce internal airflow. Since the Vector Tandem had been designed to do without skirts, it was slightly better ventilated than other human-powered vehicles, and therefore suitable for challenging endurance records.

On May 4, 1980, in one hour on Ontario Speedway's track, Ron

---

*The address of the IHPVA is Post Office Box 2068, Seal Beach, CA 90740.

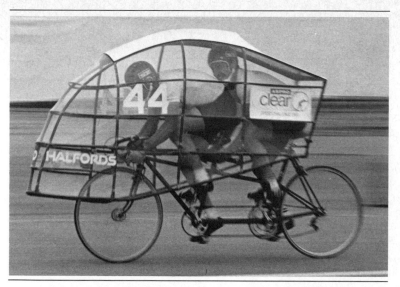

These enclosed tandem riders can attain a top speed approximately 40 percent greater than the maximum speed of a single rider crouching on a ten-speed racing bike.

PHOTO BY BUDD SYMES

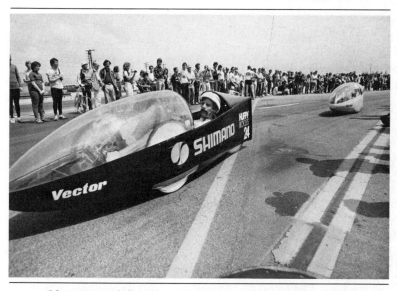

Olympic medalist Dave Grylls racing the Vector Single at an International Human-Powered Vehicles Association speed trial.

PHOTO BY BUDD SYMES

Skarin and Eric Hollander pedaled 46.30 miles aboard the Vector Tandem. Their performance compares very favorably with the 30- and 31-mile records set by Merckx and Moser on more conventional bicycles. The burning question became, What could this vehicle do on the open road?

Wilmot White of the California Department of Transportation (CALTRANS) arranged a test that sounds like every cyclist's fantasy. In 1980 CALTRANS sponsored an advanced transportation exposition at Sacramento, and White, who was also a member of the IHPVA, thought that the fair would be greatly enriched by a graphic demonstration of what human-powered vehicles could do. He suggested that the Vector Tandem be allowed to win its spurs on the one turf normally forbidden for human-powered vehicles, the freeway. CALTRANS accepted his proposal for a long-distance test of the Vector Tandem on Interstate 5—the West Coast's main north-south artery and possibly the busiest freeway on earth. Escorted by the California Highway Patrol and a caravan of CALTRANS vehicles, the Vector Tandem would leave Stockton and cover a 40-mile stretch of level interstate highway on its way to a dramatic finish at the transportation exposition.

Competitive cyclists Fred Markham and Cris Springer were recruited as the engine for the Vector Tandem's debut as a freeway cruiser. Although they were both excellent riders, neither had pedaled the Vector Tandem before, and there was a 15-mph hour crosswind on May 30, 1980, the day of the run. White says, "I was hoping they would get a little breaking in, but they only got to roll out of the parking lot about 50 feet. I cautioned them about the crosswind and told them that I thought the middle forties would be about the right pace to start out with." Under the best of conditions at the Ontario Motor Speedway, the Vector had only done 46 miles for one hour, and this trip would take the better part of an hour.

"Doggone if they didn't take off at 50 miles per hour right off the bat," recalls White, "and I thought they'd burn out for sure, but they held it all the way." They dipped as low as 45 miles per hour on the upgrades, but then accelerated to about 60 on the downgrades. In fact, one of their consistent problems was that the automobile that served as their escort vehicle was underpowered, and they occasionally were tempted to pass it. Their low-slung, aerodynamic profile made them difficult to spot from the cab of a high truck, so passing would have been ill advised. The recumbent tricycle—with its fragile external shell—might have been squashed like a June bug by some eighteen-wheeler.

The drivers of the huge rigs expressed amazement over their CB's when they realized that a human-powered vehicle was keeping pace with them on the freeway. To facilitate communication within the caravan, the Vector Tandem carried a small CB radio during the freeway trip, and Markham and Springer got to hear some of the teamsters' incredulous comments.

When the Vector arrived at the Sacramento off-ramp, the cyclists

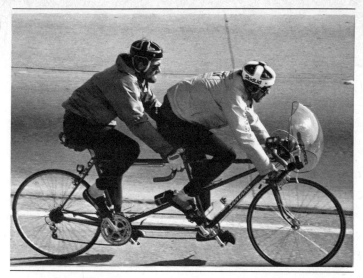

Rob Templin (left) *and Pete Penseyres* (right) *en route to the San Francisco–to–Los Angeles partially faired tandem record.* COURTESY OF GLEN BROWN

threw back their canopy to get some cool air. They had covered the 42 miles from Stockton to Sacramento at a little better than 50 miles per hour. Human-powered vehicles had proven their endurance capabilities, and Markham and Springer paid for the test in sweat.

Of late, the UCI, to its credit, has partially relented on its blanket opposition to streamlining. Aerodynamic skin suits have been common in international bicycle competition since the late 1960s. During the 1984 Olympics, track racers were permitted to use aerodynamic bicycles with such streamlined features as oval rather than round frame tubes, disk wheels, and small "funny-bike" front wheels. And, again, it should be noted that the UCI ruled in favor of Moser's record even though he used disk wheels. Although the UCI still does not separately recognize records by completely streamlined bicycles, the IHPVA more than adequately has taken up that function.

Ultralong-distance records by fully enclosed human-powered vehicles remain difficult because of the ventilation problem. However, cyclists partially protected by flexible, polystyrene windscreens have set very respectable long-distance marks. In June 1982, Jim Woodhead, riding behind a commercially available fairing called the Zzipper, covered approximately 400 miles from San Francisco to Los Angeles in 21:20. About 22 months later, Rob Templin and Peter Penseyres did the same trip on a tandem bicycle equipped with the Zzipper in a time of 19:52.51. Human-powered vehicles and partially streamlined bicycles represent a whole new frontier for the endurance athlete.

HUMAN-POWERED FLIGHT

If streamlined bicycles are on the endurance athlete's frontier, then human-powered airplanes are still in the wilderness. Leonardo da Vinci drew sketches of gliders and human-powered aircraft, but his designs remained a fantasy until the late nineteenth century. Then soaring gliders and airplanes powered by internal combustion engines made most of his dreams a reality. But, until 1977, the other part of his dream—human-powered flight—remained an unfulfilled fantasy.

In 1959, Henry Kremer, a British industrialist, offered a prize of 5,000 pounds to the first team that could produce an airworthy human-powered flying machine. (Later Kremer and others raised the ante to 50,000 pounds.) The terms of his prize were that the human-powered aircraft would have to satisfy judges appointed by the Royal Aeronautic Society that it had flown a figure-eight course approximately one mile in length.

Over the next seventeen and a half years several British, Japanese, French, West German, and American teams designed airplanes that could fly a few thousand feet under human power, but none of those planes could achieve the required turns, and none of them had gone the full distance. In general, those planes were doomed to fail because they had unfavorable weight-to-lift ratios. That is, they weighed too much to be held aloft by the area of wing that they carried. If their wings had been made larger, the internal framework of those planes would have needed strengthening to carry the additional wing structure. Hence, their weight would have increased still more. The problem of human-powered flight seemed insoluble.

Then in 1976, Paul MacCready, a champion sailplane pilot and aeronautical engineer, put together a team to build, test, and fly a human-powered aircraft. MacCready's plane was radically different from earlier designs, because it was inspired by hang-gliders. Most hang-gliders use a design patented by Francis and Gertrude Rogallo that looks like a child's toy jack. A mast protrudes perpendicularly from both surfaces of a Rogallo Wing, and guy wires are stretched from the masts to support the wings in tension. Increasing the size of a Rogallo wing does not incur the same weight penalty as increasing the size of an internally stressed wing, because the Rogallo wing has no internal support structure.

MacCready's solution of the weight-to-lift-ratio problem was a brilliant breakthrough. It required about thirteen months of experimentation, numerous low-speed crashes, and more than a few modifications to the original concept, but eventually MacCready's team built an aircraft that could accomplish far more than the short straight-line jumps of his predecessors. He had a maneuverable human-powered airplane, the *Gossamer Condor*. On August 23, 1977, Bryan Allen, a competent competitive cyclist and hang-glider pilot, pedaled the *Condor* around a 1-mile figure-eight course at Shafter Airport in California's sparsely populated, agricultural Central Valley.

Bryan Allen, who was the pilot of the airplane that won the first Kremer prize, also had ideal characteristics to be the vehicle's engine. Allen weighs 145 pounds, and though many cyclists might be able to outsprint him on the flats, he is an excellent hill climber. He has a very favorable weight-to-strength ratio for human-powered aircraft engines.

Almost before the ink was dry on the newspaper reports of MacCready and Allen's exploit, Kremer offered a new prize. It had taken seventeen and a half years for anybody to claim the first Kremer prize, and that merely required a one-mile flight. So, when Kremer announced that he would award 100,000 pounds for the first human-powered airplane that flew the 22 miles across the English Channel, it must have seemed that his prize would be unclaimed for many decades to come. MacCready and his *Gossamer* crew immediately set to work on a new plane.

After many design changes, discouraging and successful test flights, and innovations on lightweight aircraft construction, on June 12, 1979, at 04:51 Greenwich Mean Time, the *Gossamer Albatross* stood poised on a runway at Folkestone, England, ready for a first "test flight" over the English Channel. Although this "gossamer" aircraft weighed only 200 pounds without the pilot, its wingspan was 92 feet, almost half that of a Boeing 747.

Thanks to the benevolence of DuPont, the project's sponsor, the *Albatross* squadron included two planes, this one and a slightly better one that was being held in reserve for a more earnest attempt. By comparison to the earlier *Condor*, the *Albatross* was a high-tech machine built for $200,000 to compete for a prize of about $211,000. Its frame tubes were made of carbon-fiber-reinforced plastic, an exotic material. Its metal parts were limited to such essentials as sprockets, seat post, and guy wires. Its skin was gossamer-thin DuPont Mylar film. Under the scientific coaching of physiologist Joseph Mastropaolo, Bryan Allen, the successful sprinter of the first Kremer prize, had trained for the impending endurance flight.

Since they had been in England, the *Gossamer*'s pilot and its ground crew had endured six frustrating weeks waiting for suitable weather and preparing the machines and logistics for this moment. Yet, this flight was only to be a test of the equipment and the performance of the flotilla of boats that would accompany the *Albatross* on

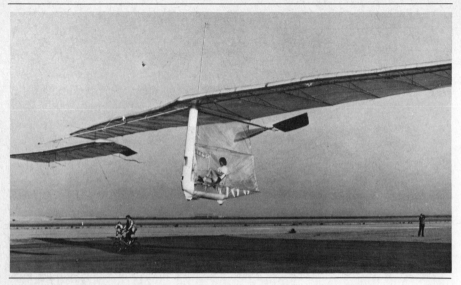

The Gossamer Albatross *with its engine, Bryan Allen,* *clearly visible.*

its low flight across the Channel. Although the press was assembled for the trial, it was not planned to fly all the way to France unless all circumstances developed favorably.

After interminable preparations, Allen launched his plane out over the Channel, and for the first time in his life the man who had logged more hours of human flight than any other man was flying over water. Although this flight was just a test run, his exhilarating takeoff filled him with optimism about the prospect of making it across the Channel on this jump.

The head wind was much stronger than desired for the flimsy craft. (The *Albatross* was designed for flight in still air.) And the transparent film covering the cockpit soon fogged up from his breathing, but Allen steadily pedaled to keep the aircraft aloft. Then he unknowingly pulled a wire loose from his radio's microphone, and though he was able to receive messages, he was no longer able to broadcast. The cause of the communication problem would not be discovered until after he landed.

During his entire flight he would have to contribute 0.3 horsepower to the drive shaft and propeller. With that energy input, a cyclist of Allen's weight and skill could propel a standard racing bicycle at 24 miles per hour in still air over level terrain. Mastropaolo had carefully tested Allen's capabilities on an ergometer—a stationary bicycle with sophisticated measuring devices. Unknown to Allen, Mastropaolo had projected the performance curves out to their limits and had pre-

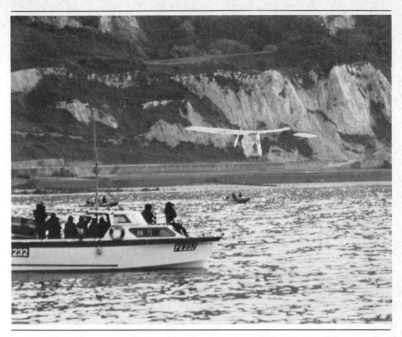

The Gossamer Albatross *leaves the Cliffs of Dover.*
COURTESY OF E. I. DU PONT DE NEMOURS AND COMPANY

dicted that the pilot could maintain his 0.3 horsepower exertion for a maximum of two hours and fifty minutes. Since it was believed that Allen could fly the plane at 10-12 knots, it was anticipated that he could cross the Channel in about two hours, a flight time well within his theoretical abilities.

Unfortunately, these predictions did not allow for the effects of air turbulence on his speed and level of exertion. At the twenty-five-minute point Allen was only 3 miles from Folkestone, and he could still see the Cliffs of Dover when he glanced backward. By one hour, he was behind schedule at 9.6 miles, and was having difficulty contributing sufficient energy to maintain altitude in the turbulent air. He had initially flown at about ten feet, but now he was dipping perilously close to the water below him. At times he had less than 1 foot altitude. If he touched the water, the attempt would be over according to the rules for the Kremer competition. After an hour and a half of flight, Allen was nearly exhausted and only two-thirds finished. He feared he could not continue the additional hour that would be necessary.

It looked as though this flight would be a trial run, after all. Allen concluded that he could not make it on this attempt. Although his flotilla of support boats was near, the noise of their engines made direct voice communication impossible, and the radio's malfunction prevented Allen from broadcasting his conclusion. When the crew below in the boats realized Allen's distress and understood that he could not send a message to them, they asked him to signal if he wanted to terminate the flight and accept a tow from the boats. Allen signaled yes.

The guide-boat crew directed him to increase his power. That would raise his altitude so the *Albatross* could be hooked from below. Despite his fatigue, Allen put on a tremendous burst of power, raising the plane to 15 feet. To his surprise, he found that it was substantially easier to fly at that altitude. He had escaped the turbulence below.

Allen changed his mind about aborting the mission, but he had no way to communicate his decision. What ensued was a cat-and-mouse game, during which the boat crew tried to catch the tow hook of the aircraft. Every time the boat crew would reach for the hook, Allen would take evasive action. Finally, the boat crew realized that he was purposely avoiding the assistance and wanted to continue the flight.

After eighteen minutes more, he ran out of water. Then two hours and ten minutes into the flight, he experienced a painful cramp in his right calf. Still he persevered and pedaled on. He favored the cramped leg and soon developed similar pain in his other leg. Finally, after thirty-five more painful minutes and several crises of motivation, he was less than a thousand yards from his destination, the beach at Cap Gris Nez. If he landed in water, no matter how shallow, he would not satisfy the terms of the Kremer competition. His easiest alternative was to crash land on rocks directly ahead of him, a messy conclusion, but one he would likely survive without injury and one that would win the prize, since the rocks were on dry land. Instead, he decided to save his airplane and turned into the wind to fly around the rocks. The turn nearly sacrificed the entire effort in a crash, but Allen regained control and put on one last powerful push, keeping his feet dry and gliding to a gentle landing on the beach. The Kremer prize belonged to the Americans of the *Albatross* squadron. The practice session turned out to be the big game.

Allen had been airborne for two hours and forty-nine minutes, just one minute less than the theoretical maximum calculated by Mastropaolo. Allen reports that when he was just 100 yards offshore he thought, "I am flying on reserves I never knew I had."

The human-powered flight across the Channel made MacCready and Allen international celebrities, but don't look for *Albatross* kits at your local sporting goods store. Fixed-wing human aircraft are too difficult to build, fly, and maintain to ever be practical or commonplace. On the other hand, it is possible to build human-powered blimps that can hover for many hours, or traverse long distances as their pilots pedal them at a pace similar to leisurely bicycling. Bryan Allen is currently involved in Bill Watson's projects to build and test human-powered blimps. Watson was a principal of the *Gossamer Albatross* construction crew and Allen is the test pilot for Watson's blimp, the *White Dwarf*. Perhaps flying those contrivances will become a sport. Blimp parks are in the offing for—you guessed it—California. Allen says that gently floating along on a pedal-powered airship is great fun. It's relatively safe too: they can't stall.

CHAPTER ▪▪▪▪▪▪▪ ▶ 5

COMBINATION EVENTS

ENDURANCE athletics used to be outside the mainstream of sport. Alan Sillitoe wrote his short story "The Loneliness of the Long-Distance Runner" as a commentary on class conflict in England, not as a treatise on the psychology of sport. The title, however, became a catchphrase applied to runners. The notion of "loneliness" seemed to say it all: long-distance runners—and by extension all endurance athletes—were brooding loners given to depressing introspection. In the public eye it was preferable for the continued development of civilization that long-distance athletes remain a monkish minority. After all, we can't tolerate too many rugged individuals cycling, swimming, or running off into the sunset.

Of course, all that was long before eighteen thousand runners ran 26.2 miles in the New York City Marathon, or a hundred thousand runners cavorted crazily through the streets of San Francisco in the Bay-to-Breakers footrace, or ten thousand cyclists rode in the RAG-BRAI (*Des Moines Register*'s Annual Great Bike Ride Across Iowa). Loneliness indeed! In 1959, when Sillitoe's story was published, few would have dared to predict mass participation in endurance athletics. Fewer still would have predicted that, just when the so-called running boom had begun to crest, the hybrid sport of triathlon would emerge and also become immensely popular.

Very quickly the triathlon became "the sport of the 1980s." It had made it big on television, and two slick magazines (*Triathlon* and *Tri-Athlete*) competed to cover it. Another publication (*Ultrasport*) serves the general endurance-sport market. Now there are even sanctioning bodies for the sport. (On the amateur side, there is the Triathlon Federation; on the professional, the Association of Professional Triathletes.) Race promoters have offered as much as $75,000 to lure the stars of the sport to televised triathlons. Bicycle, swimwear, running shoe, and beer manufacturers have enthusiastically embraced the marketing opportunities offered by the popularity of this new sport. Yet it appears, from the steady growth in triathlon participation, that this

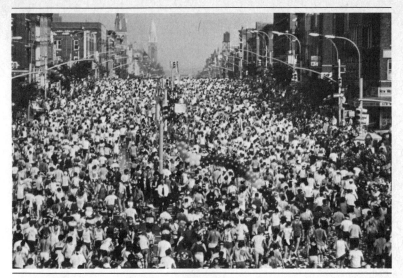

Loneliness is hardly a problem in Brooklyn, at mile 4 of the New York City Marathon. PHOTO BY DAVID CANNON

is not just another fad. *Tri-Athlete* magazine's race calendar listed 166 events between April and November 1984, and their list left out many small local triathlons and events in other countries. Each year participation increases: in 1985, according to *Triathlon* magazine, 1.1 million triathletes participated in more than twenty-one hundred triathlons. This fad probably will be a long slow burner like the Frisbee or running.

What is the origin of the triathlon? Documentation for the first triathlon seems lost in the murky past, but one thing we know for certain is that it was *not* invented by Navy Commander John Collins over a few beers with his cronies, as is frequently implied by Ironman Triathlon publicity. Clearly, the formidable Ironman in Hawaii, which includes a 2.4-mile swim, a 112-mile bike race, and a marathon footrace, is the most prestigious, best-known triathlon. Certainly it owes its origin to the naval officer's wager over a few beers. Nonetheless, the Ironman, which began in 1978, was by no means the first triathlon ever staged.

Dave Scott, who has thus far won the Ironman four times, competed in his first triathlon in 1976 in San Francisco. Low-key, casual triathlons have been conducted at San Diego's Fiesta Island at least since the early 1970s. Members of the U.S. Navy's commando unit, the SEALS (Sea, Air, and Land), have competed against each other in combined run-swim events since President Kennedy created that force in the 1960s. The Levi Strauss Ride and Tie, founded in 1970, is also a spiritual ancestor of multisports such as the triathlon because

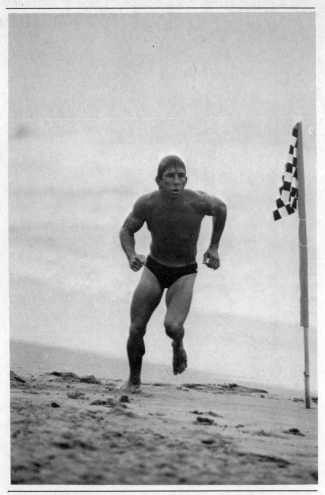

Zuma Beach lifeguard Craig "Mad Dog" Mattox takes a turn at a run-swim-run lifeguard competition.

PHOTO BY BUDD SYMES

it combines two activities, running and horseback riding (see Chapter 3). Lifeguard competitions in the United States and Australia, which in some cases date back to the 1920s, often include swim-run biathlons. The Nordic biathlon, an Olympic sport that involves marksmanship and cross-country skiing, is a multisport event that dates back many years.

One of the earliest verifiable examples of a multisport event similar to the triathlon is an individual medley completed by swim coach L. Handley in September 1901. His exertion on behalf of the Knicker- bocker and New York Athletic Clubs included six quarter-mile events: walking, running, horseback riding, bicycling, rowing, and swimming. Although he set a world record for that unconventional mile and a

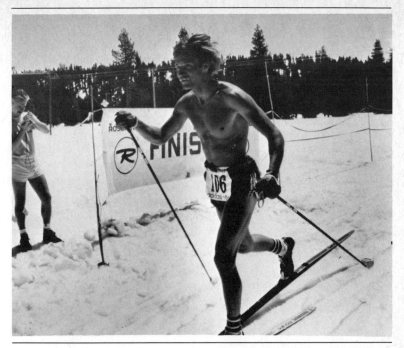

Paul Peterson finishes a run-bike-ski triathlon at Bear Valley, California, in May 1983.

PHOTO BY DAVE FREEDMAN

half, his time does not seem very impressive: fifteen minutes and forty-two seconds.

Although participation in any imaginable permutation of athletic events is worthwhile, clearly some multisport competitions are more established than others. The typical triathlon combines swimming, cycling, and running, usually in that order. In cold climes, however, winter sports may be included. For instance, the Sea Wolf Triathlon, which has been staged during freezing December weather in Anchorage, Alaska, includes a 15-kilometer cross-country ski race, a 10-kilometer run, and a 2-kilometer swim. (The swimming is at an indoor pool.) The Mountain Man Triathlon in Beaver Creek, Colorado, includes 10.96 miles of cross-country skiing, 8.5 miles of snowshoe travel, and 12.4 miles of speed skating; in all, the mountain men and women climb 6,470 feet and descend 6,910 feet to traverse 31.5 frosty miles. Racquetball, Frisbee tossing, canoeing, kayaking, weight lifting, and track-and-field contests have all been featured as part of a triathlon at one time or another. One multisport event, the Payson Golden Onion Days Pentathlon, in Payson, Utah, includes 31 miles of orienteering, in which contestants search on foot for checkpoints and the finish line by following compass courses across unmarked forested terrain.

In a little more than a decade the new sport of triathlon has passed through infancy and attained adolescence. San Diego tavern operator Tom Warren beat fifteen other participants in the second annual Ironman in 1979. But the big winner that year was the sport itself. *Sports Illustrated* ran a nine-page feature article on Warren and the Ironman contest. Media attention can quickly snowball, and ABC took its cue from *Sports Illustrated.* Since 1980, ABC's "Wide World of Sports" has covered the Ironman, and each year the number of athletes participating has increased dramatically. Thousands of would-be Ironman competitors are turned away every year, and these are serious applicants. Typically, 90 percent or more of the participants complete the race. The contestants know what they are getting into, and they train properly.

An incident at the February 1982 Ironman did more to dramatize the sport than any public relations firm ever could have wanted. In the last few feet of the marathon, women's leader Julie Moss collapsed from the exertion. Kathleen McCartney passed her, crossing the finish line first. Moss crawled to a second-place finish in the women's division. The ABC cameras kept rolling throughout the dramatic climax. Indeed, it is rumored that "Wide World of Sports" considered the Julie Moss film clip as a replacement for the crashing ski jumper, who for so many years has represented the "agony of defeat" in the show's intro. After that incident, Moss appeared on the "Today" show and in *People* magazine, and she generally became the triathlon's ambassador to the sedentary world. The main message: a wholesome, ordinary, appealing young woman, who surfed and dabbled in sports but showed no early promise of great athletic prowess, could become a champion. She could triumph personally, even if she finished second.

Most important, Julie *did* finish. She persevered and endured, providing a model for us all. The vast majority of us can't hope to finish first in such competitions, but everyone can make the all-out effort required to complete an endurance challenge.

Of course, not all triathlons are as demanding as the Ironman. There are many triple-sport events that are much shorter. The United States Triathlon Series (USTS) has gone a long way toward standardization of the triathlon. Franchised in numerous cities across America, a USTS race consists of a 1,500-meter swim, 40-kilometer bike race, and 10-kilometer run.

Still, there is some controversy about what proportion of each sport should be included in a triathlon. For instance, swimmers frequently complain that the Ironman Triathlon favors contestants with bicycling and running backgrounds. They assert that a 2.4-mile swim is not nearly as difficult as a 112-mile bike race or a 26.2-mile footrace. A champion swimmer could navigate the Ironman's 2.4 miles of open

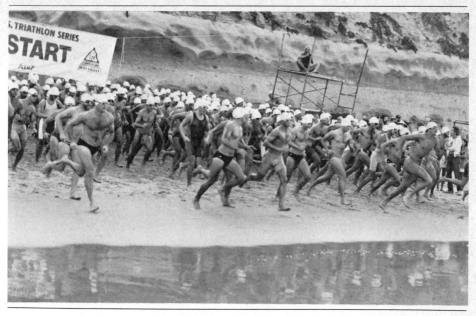

Swim start of the San Diego USTS race.

Thirty-four-year-old Jay Gehrig emerges from surf at the San Diego USTS race.

Terry Steve launches his bicycle at the San Diego USTS race.

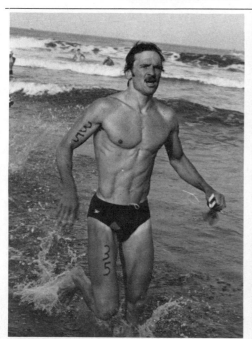

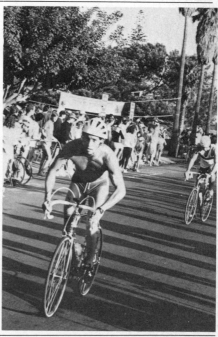

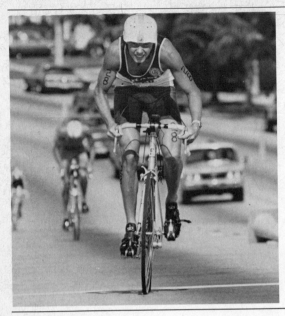
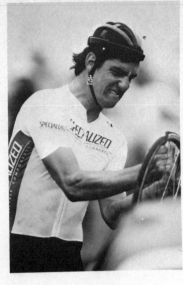

LEFT: *Standing on the pedals.*   COURTESY OF BUD LIGHT USTS

RIGHT: *Scott Molina having a bad time with a flat tire at the Malibu Triathlon. Unlike bike races, triathlons usually prohibit assistance from support crews.*

PHOTO BY BUDD SYMES

BELOW: *The bike leg of a USTS race.*

COURTESY OF BUD LIGHT USTS

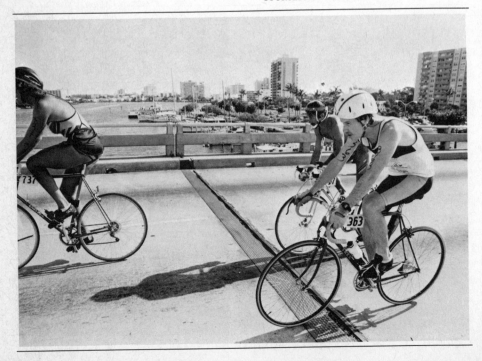

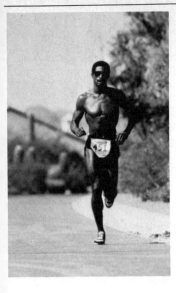

LEFT: *Keith Hill striding purposefully during the Fountain Mountain Triathlon near Phoenix, Arizona.*

PHOTO BY BUDD SYMES

BOTTOM: *Joanne Ernst finishing as number-one female.*

COURTESY OF BUD LIGHT USTS

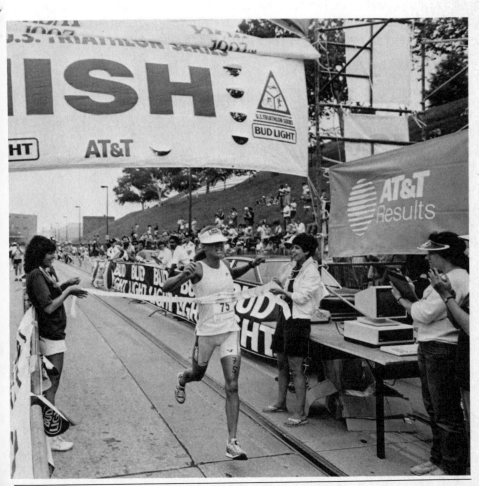

ocean in about fifty minutes, whereas a world-class cyclist might be able to blitz 112 miles in about four hours and ten minutes, and a near-record-speed marathon would take approximately two hours and ten minutes. Those who seek equity for the three sports have proposed that the lengths be adjusted so that the three events take more nearly the same amount of time. Unwilling to decrease the bike ride or foot-race, the Ironman race committee once somewhat perversely suggested that the swim be lengthened to placate the aquatic specialists. The Ironman folks polled previous participants on the question of length-ening the swim to 5 miles. Most Ironmen and women balked, so the committee retained the existing distances. Now it seems the Ironman distances are enshrined in tradition and will never be changed, although other promoters have designed races with less disproportionate race legs. An example is the aptly named Equalizer Triathlon in Lynn, Massachusetts, which has a 4-mile swim, a 50-mile bike ride, and a 15-mile run. Fletcher Hanks created the Oxford Equilateral Triathlon in Oxford, Maryland, with the goal of treating the three sports equally. Hank's event includes a 5.6-mile swim, a 20-mile run, and a 50-mile bike ride.

WHO ARE THE TRIATHLETES?

Clearly, there is no validity to the myth that triathletes are all twenty-two-year-old male lifeguards from Southern California. The prestige of triathlete's occupations in one recent Ironman Triathlon ranged from hotel bellboy to the senior crown counsel of Hong Kong, but in general they are an upscale group. In that same Ironman, 10 percent of the contestants came from the medical profession, 10 percent were executives or presidents of corporations, and 5 percent were attorneys. Ironmen and women have been students, airline pilots, fire fighters, writers, police officers, and members of the military. A goldfish in-spector from the Shimizi Goldfish Company in Hamamatsu, Japan, entered the 1983 Ironman. There even have been a few professional triathletes.

A poll by *Triathlon* magazine discovered that the median total household income of triathletes is $45,000. Sixteen percent of the participants in the 1984 USTS series were female and 84 percent were male. As to the Southern California question, it is true that the sport is popular in that region. California consistently sends the largest con-tingent to the Ironman (between 30 and 40 percent), yet, at the 1984 Ironman, contestants came from forty-six states and thirty-one coun-tries, including one Eastern-bloc nation. (Vaclav Vitovek, a thirty-one-year-old technician from Plzen, Czechoslovakia, competed in the

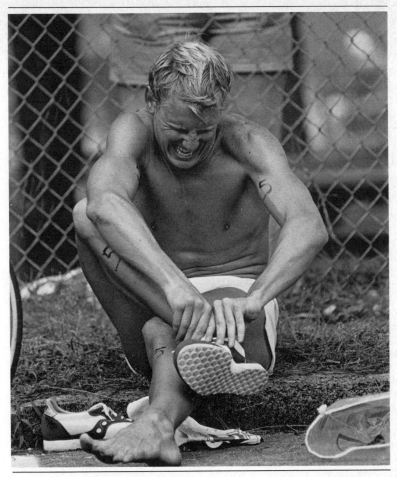

East Coast triathlete Marc Suprenant shows true grit during a transition.   COURTESY OF BUD LIGHT USTS

1984 Ironman.) Triathlons have been staged in at least fourteen different countries. There were thirty-five triathlons in Czechoslovakia during 1983; and there are now annual triathlons in France, Germany, Mexico, Guatemala, and New Zealand, to name but a few countries. The races of the 1984 United States Triathlon Series were spread out in ten cities across the breadth of America. Considering the logistical difficulties of producing a triathlon, the rapid, worldwide spread of this sport is truly remarkable.

Age is no barrier to triathlon participation. The mean age of male triathletes in 1983 was thirty-three; females, twenty-five. John Howard and Dave Scott, two very successful triathletes, are both in their thirties. Walt Stack, at seventy-three years old, completed the 1981 Iron-

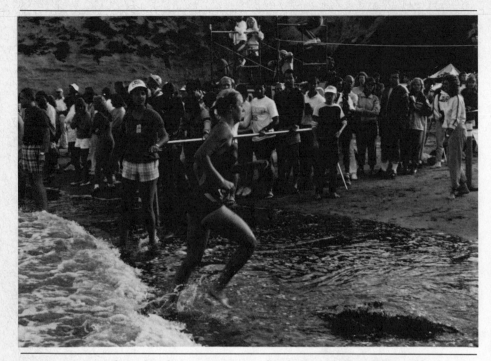

Barbara Hosking enters swim-finish chute at San Diego USTS race.   PHOTO BY ALBERT GROSS

man (26:20.25). When the Ironman imposed a minimum age standard in 1983, fifteen-year-old Rodkey Faust, who first competed at fourteen, was grandfathered into the race as the only acceptable entrant under age eighteen. Youngsters are permitted in most other triathlons, so nobody need fear being either too young or too old to enter one.

Wheelchair athletes are pursuing the sport too. The Dallas, Texas, Park and Recreation Department sponsored its first annual triathlon for the handicapped on August 13, 1983. Fourteen athletes came from throughout the United States to compete in either a long or a short version of the event. Rick Godwin of Tulsa, Oklahoma, won the long-course race, which consisted of 1.5 miles of rowing a raft, a 10-kilometer wheelchair race, and a 1-mile swim. The short-course race, whose events were half the length of the long course, was won by Ray Mathews, from Sherman, Texas.

WHY IS THE TRIATHLON SO POPULAR?

The reasons people give for becoming triathletes may explain why that new sport will be popular for a long time to come. First, for many athletes the triathlon is a logical extension of what they already do. The three most popular participation sports are bicycling, running, and swimming. When a person reaches a performance plateau in one of those three sports, or when one's sport becomes stale, it is natural to seek a new activity that broadens athletic horizons. The triathlon lets you branch out without abandoning involvement in your previous sport. Furthermore, running, swimming, and cycling are activities that most people learned during childhood. Some single-sport athletes may feel reluctant to practice new sports at which they feel they are novices, but many others who would be embarrassed to compete against more experienced athletes in an unfamiliar sport can more comfortably break into a new activity in the triathlon, where everybody is expected to lack some expertise in one or more of the events.

There are sound physiological reasons for a long-distance swimmer, runner, or cyclist to become a triathlete. Endurance sports can be rough on the body. Overtraining and overuse injuries are common, because nobody can build endurance without doing a sport a lot. Long-distance athletes are often caught in a double bind; they can't improve unless they pile on the training miles, but when they do that they are injured and then can't train at all. For many endurance athletes, a new concept, cross-training, has emerged as a way to escape over-training problems.

Cross-training is the use of a different sport to improve skill or conditioning in the principal sport. For instance, an injured runner can swim; the erstwhile world-record marathoner, Alberto Salazar, is known to do just that. Swimming maintains cardiovascular conditioning and both stresses and strengthens muscles different from the ones used for running. In the bad old days, coaches ordered their athletes to specialize, but now it is widely believed that all-around fitness improves single-sport performance.

There are two major benefits single-sport athletes obtain by doing the cross-training required for triathlons: (1) they avoid the risk of accidental injury caused by having weak and inflexible muscles not normally exercised by their principal sport, and (2) they can maintain aerobic capacity without the risk of overusing one set of muscles during training.

Triathletes also report some emotional reasons for their involvement in the new sport. Some say that they compete in triathlons because it gives them a feeling of mastery over their environment. If necessary, they know they can meet substantial physical challenges that otherwise might threaten their lives or safety. Others enter the sport because they have achieved much in their professional lives and they are seeking new challenges. The camaraderie and fulfillment of social needs is important to many triathletes; they cherish the time with their training buddies and enjoy the socializing at races. There also seems to be a pervasive reverence for one's own physical health among triathletes.

Finally, triathlete Ken Cates has given the most compelling justification for the prediction that the triathlon's current vitality will continue. With three Ironman races to Ken's credit so far, including a second-place finish in his age group (13:10), the fifty-five-year-old athlete says, "The triathlon is an everyman's race; it's accessible."

THE ATHLETES

PART

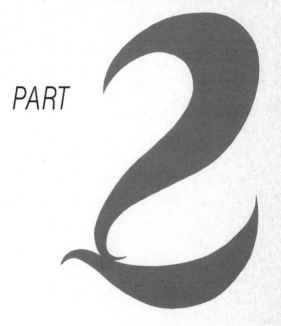

CHAPTER ▮▮▮▮▮▪▪▪ ▶ 6

THE SELF-PROPELLED

RUNNERS, walkers, and swimmers use their arms and legs to cover long distances in incredible times. What manner of creature is the self-propelled endurance athlete? Here are profiles of some specimens.

THE DEAN OF CHANNEL SWIMMERS

If we lived in a just world, the name Penny Dean would be a household word. She is not completely unknown; marathon swimming enthusiasts recognize her name. After all, her greatest endurance swimming accomplishment is comparable to Roger Bannister's historic achievement in track and field.

Penny Dean swam the English Channel on July 29, 1978, setting a record for both men and women that stands to this day. Her time of seven hours and forty minutes is the endurance swimming equivalent of running a sub-four-minute mile. In 1954, Bannister broke a human performance barrier that experts had regarded as impenetrable. Similarly, Penny Dean swam from England to France in *under* eight hours, shattering previous records; she took an hour and five minutes off the old male record and an hour and sixteen minutes off the old female record. In fact, she swam the Channel approximately twenty minutes faster than her diesel-powered guide boat was able to convey her back to England.

Sebastian Coe, Steve Cram, and other runners who came after Bannister gradually pushed the time for the mile down below 3:47. Many sports observers believe that breaking a critical barrier, such as the four-minute mile, inspires subsequent records, which make the old milestone seem a mediocre achievement. As these words are written, in the spring of 1985, it seems that Penny Dean's durable Channel mark is an exception to that rule. Perhaps during an upcoming Channel-swimming season—only July and August offer warm enough water—some swimmer will break the seven-year-old record. World professional swimming champion Paul Asmuth took two shots at it in the summer of 1985. He was the most serious contender in recent years, but he failed each time by more than half an hour.

Whoever finally exceeds her standard will be one hell of a swimmer. Penny says, "I swam the whole Channel like a 200-meter sprint in the Olympics." Her pace never went below 85 strokes per minute and often was up to 93. Dean is a prime example of the new breed of swimmer, those who have dominated endurance ocean swims since the late 1970s. With skills and a rapid pace developed by speedwork in swimming pools, they have replaced earlier swimmers who specialized in slow long-distance ocean swimming.

Penny Dean's highly esteemed navigator, the late Reg Brickell, boat captain for numerous Channel swims, was amazed by her performance. Had he fully comprehended her capabilities he probably would have delayed departure by two hours so that Penny would have approached the French coast during more favorable tide conditions. Although Penny had timidly asked what would happen if she were within striking distance by seven hours, Brickell simply didn't believe that was possible and predicated the plans on the assumption that she would be within a few miles by nine hours. As they approached the coast of France the tide was pulling her away from Cap Gris Nez, and she had to redouble her efforts to avoid missing her landfall. If she hadn't bulldozed through the tide to make the landing at Cap Gris Nez, she would have been pulled many miles up the coast, lengthening the swim by hours.

At present, Dean philosophically accepts the relative lack of recognition for her moment of glory. She says, "I expected my life to change. I expected the world to stand still and then begin rotating around me, but hardly anybody noticed at all." Penny grew up in Santa Clara, California, and she had trained with that city's prestigious club, which has spawned numerous Olympic swim champions. Her hometown *did* declare October 17, 1978, Penny Dean Day. Penny, unfortunately, could not afford the fare from Los Angeles to Santa Clara and thus missed the festivities. Penny recalls, "At first I was bitter about the things that didn't happen, but now I accept it better."

This is more than an example of endurance sport playing second fiddle to the so-called major sports. True, Dean wasn't vying for a Heisman trophy, but she was nonetheless playing in the big leagues. The world does sometimes pay homage to marathon swimmers. In 1875, for example, Matthew Webb required nearly triple the time of Penny Dean to become the first conqueror of the Channel, but he was rewarded by international acclaim and a sum of money that, when corrected for inflation, would amount to about $250,000 today. Trudy Ederle, who in 1926 became the first woman to breach the English

Channel, was honored by a ticker-tape parade in New York and remained a celebrity for the balance of her life. Florence Chadwick and Greta Anderson, female Channel swimmers of the 1950s and 1960s, have greater name recognition today than our contemporary Penny Dean, who has set a remarkably impressive speed record.

Considering what she did, Penny Dean's aspirations for recognition were reasonable, but unfortunately, at the age of twenty-three, she was not savvy enough about self-promotion to make her dream of glory come true. Short-distance Olympic swimmers such as Johnny Weismuller, Esther Williams, and Mark Spitz have done very well financially. Other endurance swimmers, of lesser—though still impressive—ability, have capitalized far better than Penny on their swimming accomplishments. In 1978, Diana Nyad—a fine long-distance swimmer—attempted to swim from Cuba to the United States inside an antishark cage towed by a boat. She was not able to successfully complete her swim, yet her publicity, which utterly eclipsed the coverage of Penny Dean's swim that same year, led to a lucrative career as a television sports commentator. Penny's only prize for the Channel swim was the Rolex watch awarded by the Channel Swimming Association for the fastest crossing of the summer.

Actress Julie Ridge accomplished one of her most important personal goals when she made it to Broadway as a star of *Oh! Calcutta!!* Since then Ridge has also swum the English Channel (17:55), and has become the first person to do a 56-mile double circumnavigation of Manhattan Island. Julie says she is embarrassed that she has received so much more publicity for her swims than have some much faster endurance swimmers. Of course, in the acting trade publicity is essential, so she needs the press. *Life* magazine published her diary and illustrated the article with a photo of Julie and her pet snake, but Julie laments that so far the notoriety has not translated into acting or athletic opportunities that would erase the debts she incurred to finance her endurance activities. (Julie Ridge sought corporate sponsorship for her swims, but her role in the "erotic" musical comedy *Oh! Calcutta!!* more or less precluded support by the image-conscious companies she approached.)

Penny Dean has adjusted admirably to the disappointment of not cashing in on her sport. A key to that adjustment can be found in her motivations to swim the Channel in the first place. She had resolved to swim the Channel when she was ten years old, after attempting a swim across San Francisco's Golden Gate.

Although the entrance to San Francisco Bay is only a mile or so wide at low tide, the cold water and heavy maritime traffic can make the Golden Gate swim a particularly treacherous undertaking. At certain points in the tide cycle, swimming across is impossible because water rushes out of the bay at 9 knots, a current strong enough to sweep Moby Dick along in its path, not to mention a ten-year-old girl.

Her coaches, Ray and Zada Taft, had contrived the highly publicized swim of the Golden Gate as a demonstration that even children can be immunized against drowning if you teach them to swim. The coaches wanted little Penny to become the youngest female to cross from San Francisco to Marin. She was accompanied by eight-year-old Bruce Farley. Unfortunately, the pair of youngsters had to stop several times and tread water while merchant ships entered the harbor. Penny was chilled by the inactivity of those interminable delays, and she gave in to temptation when her overcompassionate support team invited the shivering child to climb aboard the boat and quit the swim. Her companion Bruce swam the remaining 400 yards to the Marin shore to become the youngest male to swim the Golden Gate.

Penny was devastated that her mother was not on the pier to greet her when she arrived by boat. She believed that her mother's absence was a disapproving expression of parental disappointment. The ten-year-old silently vowed to compensate for that failure by someday swimming the English Channel.

Penny's relationship with her mother, Frances Dean, has been a key element in her athletic career. It was her mother who regularly took the adolescent to and from swim practices at the Santa Clara Swim Club. (Penny began swimming before she was one year old, and attended daily training sessions from the age of six.) Later, as an intercollegiate swimmer, Penny says, "I would call my mother from school to get a kick in the pants if my motivation to train was lagging." Frances Dean flew to England several weeks before the Channel swim and walked the rocky beach of Folkestone, counting Penny's stroke rate as she trained in the chill and choppy water beyond the harbor.

It was not until thirteen years after the Golden Gate fiasco, when Penny attained her goal in the Channel, that she finally learned her mother's reason for leaving the dock in California. Frances Dean was surprised to read her daughter's interpretation of the incident in the draft of an autobiography Penny had written. She explained that she had left the pier because she feared she had put too much pressure on Penny to achieve athletically.

In any case, Penny's goal to compensate for her early "failure" has been more than amply fulfilled. Along the way Penny has earned a degree in history from Pomona College and a master's degree in physical education. She successfully competed intercollegiately in the pool and trained in the ocean as much as thirteen hours a day. En route to her triumph in European water she set records for both the

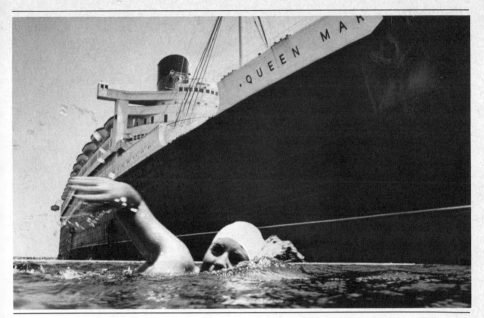

Penny Dean training in Long Beach Harbor, California.
PHOTO BY HARALD JOHNSON

single and double crossing of the channel between Catalina Island and the California coast. (The round trip is 42 miles.) Three times she swam in the Junior National Long Distance Championships, winning that 3-mile event in 1971. Later she also competed in two AAU Nationals. This is not the profile of a quitter or a failure.

People often have the misconception that champion athletes are somehow different from the rest of us; that their training is unhampered by the mundane matters that concern everybody else. Penny says she had the same day-to-day problems that plague all people. Her car was just as likely as anybody else's to break down or have a flat on the freeway. Her swimming skills didn't immunize her to either emotional traumas or colds. She fell in and out of love with boyfriends just like other young women. She took her schoolwork seriously and had to turn in the same assignments as all the other students. She had to figure out how to pay her bills and study and train at the same time. Her friends sometimes let her down and sometimes were right there when she needed them. She got tired and felt lonely and lost heart for the enterprise on more than one occasion.

For a long time Penny was completely unaware of one other problem that made her swimming difficult and even might have threatened her life. From the earliest days of her swimming career Penny experienced pain in her left shoulder and arm. She attributed this pain to benign training soreness, and doctors at first misdiagnosed the problem as tendinitis or bursitis. When her arm began to turn blue a few months before the Channel swim, Penny sought medical attention. (At the time she was training and competing in Europe on a Watson Foundation fellowship, which also financed her Channel assault.) A Swiss heart specialist determined that she suffered from a rare congenital defect; she had been born without an anterior artery in her left arm. The posterior artery, which was supplying all the blood to Penny's left arm, was now being blocked by muscle development as a result of her training. She was cutting off circulation every time she raised her arm above her shoulder; that is, every stroke was causing painful damage.

Although her physician warned that continued swimming could put her arm in jeopardy of amputation, Penny had gone too far toward her goal to quit then. She did the Channel swim in spite of excruciating pain during the final few miles. Subsequently, an operation, which broke new medical ground, has reduced the constriction of the posterior artery in her left arm. But a recent series of mild strokes has suspended Penny's swimming career. The Roger Bannister of endurance swimming is forbidden by her doctor to train, and possibly she will never be able to resume long-distance swimming.

A second key to Penny's adjustment to the lack of recognition is the way she leads her life. She feels she has a duty to give something back to the sport of swimming. She has joined the faculty of her alma mater, Pomona College, where she teaches a course in the philosophy and history of sport; she also coaches water polo and swimming. Watching her at work, it is obvious that she is dedicated to the well-being of the athletes she trains. She says, "I have to be their coach, their friend, their sister, and sometimes their mother." Penny aspires to break into the "old-boy network" by becoming the first female coach of the U.S. Olympic swim team.

Penny is also a founder of the Catalina Channel Swimming Federation. That organization sanctions and encourages swims across the body of water that was first conquered on January 15, 1927, after chewing-gum king William Wrigley, Jr., put up a $25,000 prize for a race. He wanted to promote his chewing gum and the development of the island as a resort. His call for entries was answered by eighty-seven men and fifteen women.

That first Catalina race, which has been called "the most spectacular event in aquatic sports," was won by seventeen-year-old Canadian national swim champion George Young. In marked contrast to Penny Dean's English Channel swim, fifteen thousand spectators greeted Young on his emergence from the water. For hours spectators had been flashing their car lights to show him the way to the beach. His progress was monitored by KNX radio. Upon his arrival the sky was lit with pyrotechnics. Young swam the Catalina Channel in 15:44.30.

Young and a friend had worked their way to California from Toronto, at first riding a secondhand motorcycle with sidecar, but hitchhiking after the machine broke down beyond repair in Little Rock, Arkansas. Trudy Ederle, who was still quite a celebrity due to her English Channel swim, declined to enter the event, but she advised the contestants, "If you feel like quitting, just keep right on swimming anyway." Nobody other than George Young obeyed her instruction. He had received the same admonition about finishing what he started from his mother, a hearty, penniless invalid who had invested her meager savings of $135 to help the boy make the trip. As the only finisher among the 102 entrants, he surely deserved his prize. However, his agent, Henry O'Bryne, who had financed Young's final preparations, ended up with 40 percent of the prize money.

Since the Wrigley extravaganza, no comparable endurance swim race has been staged. The picture that begins to emerge from all this is one of a sport in which the financial rewards are usually meager or are carted off by somebody other than the athletes. At best, marathon swimmers are treated capriciously and inconsistently. Although there is a professional marathon swimming circuit that provides modest prize money for a few, the true rewards must still come from within the swimmers.

THE KEY TO ULTRAMARATHON RUNNING

Timothy Joseph Key—T.J. to his friends—takes great pride in completing the ultradistance runs he enters. He says that he once was a quitter, but running is one thing he has been able to complete. Actually, T.J. has achieved other conventional measures of success, but his past is strewn with self-inflicted adversity and failure, and running has been an essential strategy in reversing that pattern.

Born in 1944 on an Indian reservation near Rosebud, South Dakota, T.J.'s early childhood included wholesome, pleasant outdoor activity. Although he is not an Indian, he hunted and fished with the Indian boys of his own age and at first showed no signs of the delinquency and violence that would soon envelop his life. When his father's milk delivery business went sour, the Keys moved from the rural Badlands to urban San Diego, California.

In San Diego, T.J. began to get into trouble. Undiagnosed vision problems set back his education, and by his late teens he was far more likely to be seen in a pool room than a schoolroom. Brawling in the local bars became a way of life for young T.J. He eventually quit school altogether. At eighteen years old, he and a friend, Jim Hammond, ran away from their problems, hitchhiking and bumming their way around the country until they were arrested for vagrancy in Las Vegas. While in jail, T.J. was charged with a murder in Los Angeles that he could not possibly have committed. At the time of the crime he was in northern Montana, working as a migrant wheat harvester, but he was powerless to prove his innocence and was never allowed to get an attorney or even make a phone call. When somebody else was finally arrested and charged with the murder, T.J. was released with a stern warning to get out of town and never return.

More wanderings, more low-life, and a short career of petty theft followed. He and a companion from home, John Bruckner, were caught burglarizing a grocery store in Key West, Florida. Time on the county work gang followed, but he and Bruckner were made trusties by the guards, who liked them and treated them with the same casual goodwill that they displayed toward long-term Key West citizens. They responded to the loose supervision by simply walking away from their sentence. Surprisingly, they were never listed as fugitives. T.J. explains, "Things were relaxed and friendly in Key West, everybody there knew everybody else, and most people came from families that had lived on the key for hundreds of years. They had accepted us as locals." After their "escape," T.J. and John contended with the harsh street life in Miami and Detroit for a few months and then bummed their way back to San Diego.

It was 1966, and the Vietnam War was in full swing. In T.J.'s absence, increasingly threatening draft notices had been piling up at his parents' house. To avoid more jail time, T.J. responded to the army's call. His high score on the army aptitude test revealed that he was not the imbecile he and just about everybody else had supposed. Despite his educational deficiencies, he was offered an opportunity to attend officer candidate school. He declined that opportunity, partly because he would have incurred several years' more obligation to the army, and partly because fresh-baked second lieutenants were known to have a high mortality rate in Vietnam. Nonetheless, he volunteered for an army position in the navy's Underwater Demolition Team (UDT) training.

T.J. was on his way to duty as a frogman. He excelled at the rigorous commando training, which included long runs and ultralong swims. On nighttime swims, the UDT trainees were released from submarines and had to find the unseen shore with the aid of a map and compass. In spite of the hazardous combat duty that might await him, it looked like T.J. was finally succeeding at something. But he managed to snatch defeat from the jaws of victory.

Those were the days of draft resistance and anti–Vietnam War sentiment. Morale in the U.S. Army was low, and for many draftees counting days was a major pastime. Other than the "lifers"—the career soldiers, whom the conscripts despised—virtually everybody else in the army had a "short-timer's calendar" on which he marked how many days and hours of service remained. As graduation from UDT school approached, T.J. had only a few months of service left. If he graduated, his military obligation would be extended. He purposely flunked the written final exam. He was glad to shorten his army career, but deep inside he regretted that he had quit again. He had wanted to be a frogman, but somehow he had lacked the ability to delay gratification by serving a little longer in order to attain a cherished goal. He was not willing to pay the required price for success. With yet another humiliating failure behind him, T.J. marked time for the short remainder of his army stint.

The self-imposed label of "quitter" had taken control of T.J.'s life. Back home after military service, he decided to finish his high school education in adult school, but once more he quit before achieving his goal. He later returned to the high school program, and this time he succeeded despite himself. The school's principal, who had known T.J. and his problems when he was in regular high school, showed compassion. After the second time T.J. quit adult school before graduating, the principal bent the rules. A totally unexpected high school diploma arrived at T.J.'s house by mail. Finally, a break.

As a veteran, T.J. was entitled to Veteran's Administration educational benefits; he decided to continue his schooling in a local community college. At first his drinking and brawling made it seem that college would be yet another failure to add to his long list, but somewhere along the line he got hold of himself and radically reformed his life. Carousing at the bars and watching television dropped from his repertoire, and he became a dedicated student. He supplemented his meager veteran's benefits by buying used refrigerators, fixing them up, and selling them at a profit. Then he discovered the volatile Southern California real estate market.

By finagling for loans—occasionally falsifying the employment information on finance applications—T.J. was able to purchase dilapidated houses and rental units. He would fix them up and try to keep them rented, while he subsisted marginally in order to meet his loan payments. It was a juggling act, but by 1977 the young man who had previously quit or failed at everything else was able to liquidate some of his holdings and gain enough equity to live comfortably, though in a somewhat austere style.

Meanwhile, many of T.J.'s early acquaintances were either languishing in jail or had died young from their alcoholism, drug abuse, and violent activities. By contrast, somehow, at age thirty-three, T.J.

had emerged from the gutter financially secure, and the proud possessor of a B.A. in sociology from San Diego State University. He was modestly wealthy and wise, but unfortunately he wasn't also healthy. The once muscular and athletic youngster now stood on the threshold of middle age at least forty pounds overweight and a good candidate for lung cancer; he was a three-pack-a-day smoker. Nonfilter Camels, at that!

Feeling that he had paid for his success with his health, T.J. resolved to become fit again. He began running on the track at San Diego State University. At first he could barely make it once around the quarter-mile oval, but gradually his endurance returned. He stopped smoking, for once quitting something for the correct reason. He started training with the distance runners on the university's track team, although he typically finished the roadwork long after those young competitors had showered and left the gym. Then he entered the 1977 Mission Bay Marathon, which he finished in a time of 3:30. Several months followed during which he ran a marathon somewhere every single weekend. His average weekly mileage rose to 130, and even 210 one week. He lowered his marathon time to 2:38.

T.J.'s new avocation became an integral part of his renaissance. He had shown himself and the world that he didn't have to be a loser, and the long footraces became a personal metaphor of his improving self-esteem. Says T.J., "It's meant a lot to me in a lot of ways, because before in my life I quit just about everything I started. Then, when I found out I could actually do things, complete them and feel good about them, there was no stopping me. I started to live at thirty-five just because of that." Running was more evidence of success.

Then T.J. heard about the Western States 100-Miler, the trail run from Squaw Valley to Auburn, California, across the rocky and often snowy crest of the Sierra Nevada Mountains. The marathon had by then become routine for him. Since he was doing the mileage to support it, he entered some 50-mile and 100-mile track races to train for the Western States. He ran the Western States race in 1979, finishing the course in a time of 21:45. T.J. had become an ultramarathoner.

Next T.J. and a running buddy, Tommie Jackson, got the crazy idea to go after the twenty-four-hour, two-man relay record. Jackson and Key trained several months for the record attempt. Through trial and error they developed a reasonable strategy. The plan was to run at about a seven-minute-mile pace the entire twenty-four hours. They calculated that at that rate they would run more than 200 miles, exceeding the previous record by at least 12 miles. On November 24, 1980, Jackson and Key were on a track at Carlsbad, California, along with a score of other teams. They were the only team that had only two runners; most of the others had ten.

Early in the relay race, their plans began to go awry. Jackson was feeling frisky—too frisky—and he was running some of the early miles at a 5:50 pace. His average was down around 6:10 minutes per mile. He would run several fast miles and pass off the baton in order to sit down while T.J. ran several more miles at a moderate pace. T.J. then would pass back the baton, and Jackson would get up and sprint again. The problem was all the stopping and starting—sitting down and getting up again. T.J. says, "When you do that you tend to freeze up. Rigor mortis sets in after ten or twelve hours. I avoided sitting more than three minutes at any time during the entire twenty-four hours."

Because they were only seeing each other to exchange the baton, T.J. and Tommie could not confer with each other on strategy, and their handlers were relatively powerless to counsel Tommie to practice moderation. He felt strong and was going fast, so how could they make him slow down? Wasn't speed the objective?

Unfortunately, a tortoise strategy is often wiser than a hare strategy in ultradistance running. T.J. recalls, "After twelve hours Tommie began to hit the wall. He hit the wall so hard he was down to 9-minute miles, and the handlers had to pull him out of the chair to get him back on the track."

Then the worst happened. Years after the event, the anguish still shows on T.J.'s face as he recounts, "I came around one time to hand off to him, and he wasn't there. He was gone. There was a motor home next door, right off the track, and the handlers said, 'He's in there.' I walked over with the baton. I walked in. Everybody was standing around, and he was lying there with his eyes shut. He looked like dead meat. They were all going, 'He's had it.' "

Describing a scene reminiscent of the film *They Shoot Horses, Don't They?* T.J. continues: "We looked at each other. I said, 'Tom, you gotta do one thing: take this baton, go out there, and walk around the track one time; that's all you gotta do. I don't care if you do anything else. Just do it once.' I handed him the baton; he got up. He had sworn to the people, before I walked in there, that he wasn't getting up, but he did what I said. He walked a mile in about twenty minutes, so I started running 6:20's and 6:10's. We're talking about thirteen hours into this, but I had to pick up the pace to make up the slack."

Tommie kept going. He continued walking. T.J. says, "He got to the point where he could walk two laps and run two laps. He was doing eight- to eight-and-a-half-minute miles at seventeen hours into it." At twenty hours, both the runners were doing seven-minute miles. They had returned from the dead.

T.J. explains, however, that his mid-race sprinting took its toll toward the end: "I started slowing down, and he was in better shape

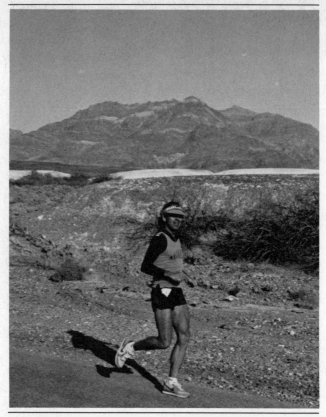

T. J. Key at the Death Valley Hundred Mile Invitational
COURTESY OF DEE KOHLER

than I was. My last mile was at a nine-minute pace. I totally ran myself into the ground. Complete exhaustion. I was wiped out for days."

Jackson and Key broke the existing two-man, twenty-four relay record by 6 miles. They ran 193.75 miles, falling short of their 200-mile goal.

The sport of ultramarathon running has blossomed since 1980. There are many more opportunities to run long races than there used to be, and many of those races are set in exotic locales. One of T.J.'s great dreams is to compete in a cross-U.S. race, reminiscent of the corn-and-bunion derbies of the 1920s. Both Jackson and Key now favor running in the scenic, rugged mountains to running around a monotonous cinder track. Three years in a row T.J. ran Colorado's Pike's Peak Marathon, an ascent to 14,000 feet, followed by a bone-jarring descent back to the bottom. He says, "When you hit the wall at Pike's Peak you don't get up and go on."

According to T.J., "On the track you're too much like a machine." For contrast, he describes trail running: "You're out there, and sometimes you're alone for hours in the wilderness, and it can be a real adventure." T.J. rhapsodizes, "I've fallen in love with trail running." So much in love that he ran the 1984 Western States 100-Miler, despite a swollen leg that kept him in bed until shortly before the race. The swelling was a consequence of a mishap on a training run six weeks earlier; a rattlesnake had bitten his leg. Indeed, it *can* be a real adventure.

Key has sought running adventures in some out-of-the-way venues. He once spent several weeks running in the desolate tribal lands of the Tarahumara Indians in Chihuahua, Mexico. This is an area of Mexico that is so remote that it isn't accessed by any paved roads. Autos must contend with primitive dirt roads. The railroad connection wasn't completed until the 1960s. There are few outposts at which to buy provisions, so T.J. pretty much lived off the land on this two-week adventure run. He carried a few meager supplies in a fanny pack.

He had hoped to meet the Tarahumara Indians, because they are an almost legendary tribe of runners for whom running has a spiritual and cultural significance. Contacting them was not difficult; they are everywhere in that isolated region.

The traditional culture of the tribe has been disrupted adversely by the tourism that accompanied the railroad's intrusion. However, many of the Tarahumara are still self-sufficient practitioners of subsistence agriculture. They cultivate small plots near the huts and caves in which they live just as their ancestors had a thousand years before. The Tarahumara are easily distinguished from other citizens of Mexico, because they have not intermarried with non-Indians. Their culture is closer to that of Indians in isolated areas of U.S. Indian reservations than it is to the culture of the majority of Mexicans.

T.J. reminisces about his experience in Mexico: "I'd be running through those canyons, and I would see them, and they would yell at me across the canyons. I don't know what they were yelling, but it was always good, you know, it made me feel good, and I'd yell back at them. They love to run, and some of those people would be running; but it wasn't like they were doing races. They have a game they play; they kick this little round wooden ball for a day or two at a time. Whole tribes go on these runs, families and everything. They seem to maintain about a seven-minute pace. For some people that would be running; for other people it wouldn't. Considering the elevation, anywhere from seven to ten thousand feet, I'd call it running."

According to T.J., folklore in our own modern tribe of ultradistance runners has it that the Tarahumara were recently invited to send entrants to a marathon somewhere in the Midwest. The tribal elders considered the invitation and then inquired about the distance involved in our running ceremony. They were told it was 26.2 miles. For that trivial distance the Tarahumara deemed it sufficient to send two of their very young girls.

Even among ultradistance runners, for whom the extraordinary is common place, T. J. Key is recognized as a master of the craft. He was one of the founders of the San Diego Ultra-Distance Society (SDUDS). At first that club was a rather informal association whose purpose was to permit four or five guys to train together and carpool to the out-of-town races. At one of these out-of-town races, the American River 50-Miler in northern California, an incident occurred that changed the name of the club. The members had been more or less satisfied with the original name (because SDUDS could be mispronounced "studs" if you slurred your speech a little). Nonetheless, the new name was earned in a race, so it has stuck.

The incident? A SDUDS member, Mike Wade, was running on a particularly rutted section of the 50-mile trail when he caught up with a group of runners who came from the communities near the race course. Those runners readily included Wade in their small talk, although the others all knew each other and seemed to have a proprietary attitude toward the American River Trail. Mistaking Mike Wade for a "local" like themselves, one of the group commented to him, "I don't know why all those flatlanders from L.A. and San Diego come up here and run in our races; they're wasting their time. They'll never even finish." Wade replied, "Well, I'm from San Diego, and I'll see you guys later." Then he took off, leaving the locals in the dust.

The club's name was changed to the Flatlanders. Considering that the Flatlanders mostly run in the mountains, the members felt their new name had a pleasingly ironic ring to it. With the new name came some new members, and some formal organization. The members instituted regular meetings, a newsletter, club dinners, a schedule of trail races sponsored by the club, and affiliation with The Athletics Congress (TAC).

The entry requirements established for the Flatlanders make it one of the most exclusive organizations in sports. To become a Flatlander you have to run a 100-mile race in a time of less than twenty-four hours and be elected to membership by a two-thirds majority vote of the current members. The membership base is no longer limited to the San Diego region; it has become national, even international, in scope.

To retain your Flatlander membership you must run a 100-miler in under twenty-four hours every eighteen months. As T.J. puts it, "We don't want to carry around any dead weight." Over one hundred ultradistance runners have achieved Flatlander membership over the years, although the continuing membership roster hovers at around forty or so lean-and-mean zealots who satisfy the requirement for a century run once every year and a half.

T. J. Key, who once considered himself a quitter and failure, turned his life around and became an endurance athlete. Other ultradistance runners recognize his mastery of the sport; his fellow Flatlanders elected him the first president of their club.

WALK, DON'T RUN

Penny Dean began her athletic career at one year old, when she was first taught to swim. She was training intensely for her sport by the age of six. She was groomed and encouraged to become a competitive swimmer throughout her youth. In short, she was born and raised to be an athlete. At the other extreme, T. J. Key was born to raise hell and finally became an endurance athlete instead. For him the route to endurance sport was a logical extension of his personal struggle to make his life amount to something.

There are many different trails up the same mountain. Dale Sutton (a dentist) and Lizzy Kemp (a student majoring in physical education) are two endurance athletes who discovered their sport in a manner totally different from both Penny and T.J.

Sutton and Kemp are long-distance racewalkers, and both of them have followed the path of least resistance into that uncommon sport. Dale Sutton and Lizzy Kemp are Flatlanders, but they qualified for that exclusive club by walking rather than running 100 miles in under twenty-four hours. As Dale says, "It's really neat to blow by a runner. Walking is a lot harder than running, because when you're running and you get tired you can walk; but if you're walking and you get tired, what do you do?"

Racewalking is different from conventional walking. Racewalkers must lock their knees on each step and, unlike runners, must have one foot in contact with the planet at all times. The movement of a racewalker is analogous to that of the trotter in Thoroughbred horse racing. If you break into a run you are disqualified. Lizzy Kemp says, "When you are walking you fantasize about running, because you are so sick of having to lock your knees." But she explains that she racewalks because "it's less injurious and has more of a social aspect." Lizzy believes that in racewalking "the big contest between Dale and me is over who can eat the most and who can talk the most."

Lizzy Kemp also believes that her sport is more difficult than running. She explains: "Running you use about 40 percent of your body, because your arms pretty much just hang out. Really, your legs

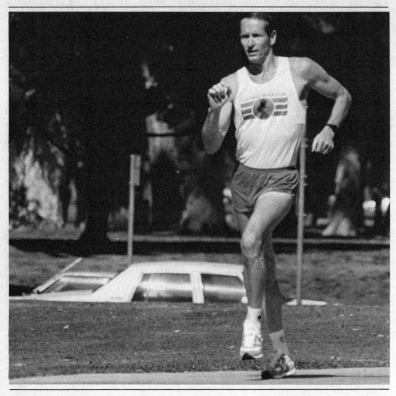

Racewalker Dale Sutton, D.D.S.

just hang out too, because they're floating. They're not going into position. But with racewalking you use at least 60 percent of your body—your back, your arms, your waist, your feet, your ankles. Running, you use primarily the thigh and calf. Racewalking, you use both sides of your legs. Your shins, your hamstrings, and your butt muscles get real developed, whereas with running that doesn't happen."

Dale Sutton recalls his earliest exposure to racewalking: "I had never walked a step in my life, although I had seen it in movies." Then he saw the 50-kilometer Olympic racewalk on television. Soon after, he tried racewalking himself: "A day or two later, there was a masters track meet, so I entered the 100-meter sprint. Well, I'm always *not bad* in a sprint; I can beat most guys. So I entered the thing. In this race was John Carlos, Pete Smith, and two French guys from the Olympics. They did about 10.1 for 100 meters. I did a 13 flat. Those people looked really little from my vantage when they crossed the finish line. I was last. I mean *last!* At the same meet they had a 3,000-meter racewalk. So I decided, 'Well shoot, let's give that a try.' I put myself at the back of the pack. The event started. I had no previous experience, so I emulated the other walkers, and I went around the course. I didn't know you weren't supposed to talk to them, but I asked the racewalking judge, 'How am I doing?' He said, 'You're looking good.' I said, 'Am I legal?' He said, 'Yeah, terrific.' The thought went through my mind, 'If I'm looking good, and I'm legal, how come we're going so gol-danged slow?' I decided to pick up the pace, and I went to the front of the pack. People were looking at me: 'What the heck's he doing?' I continued my escalation of pace, and before long I had lapped the whole field. I averaged around nine minutes a mile for 3,000 meters, which isn't very fast by today's standards, but I lapped the field, and I won a gold medal. So at that point I figured, I am the absolute slowest of the fast guys, and I'm the fastest of the slow guys.''

Dale explains how he followed the course of least resistance into a new sport: "Because I'm good at racquetball and wrestling, I do those. I'm bad at Ping-Pong, so I never play Ping-Pong. Having had no instruction, I just tried to emulate what I saw, and evidently I was a natural racewalker.''

Lizzy Kemp was a natural racewalker too, but in her case it took a second try to discover that. Reminiscing about her introduction to the sport, she says, "I feel that people tend to like what they're good at. I've always gone for being famous. I used to be into acting and singing, and I used to do singing telegrams for a living. Then a friend of mine, Adriane Hughes, said, 'Hey let's go down to Mission Bay Park [San Diego]. I'll show you how to racewalk.' I had always dabbled a little bit in athletics. I had played field hockey in high school, I did aerobics, I ran. But I didn't do any of it every day seriously. I went out and racewalked with Adriane. It was so hard, I hated it.''

If Adriane had been less persistent, Lizzy very likely would not have discovered the hard-core racewalker that lurked within her dilettante's body. She now believes that the first experience had been difficult because they had walked at race pace and she didn't have the muscles for that. For two weeks after that first attempt Lizzy studiously ignored the new sport. Then Adriane asked Lizzy how the racewalking was going and invited Lizzy to accompany her and a group, which included Dale Sutton, on a workout in the park. Lizzy didn't want to admit she hadn't been training, so she went along. This time everyone racewalked at a social pace, and Dale noticed that Lizzy had a smooth, graceful style. She was a natural.

Lizzy began to train regularly. By November 1981 she felt proficient enough to pace Dale Sutton for the first 50 miles of a 100-mile track race. That race was The Athletics Congress 100-Mile Racewalking Championship. At the 50-mile point, where she had originally planned to stop, Lizzy still felt good, so she just kept on going. Before she knew what had happened, the neophyte racewalker had clicked off 75 miles and was beginning to attract attention from the observers.

Because she had not really intended to finish the race, Lizzy had not bothered to arrange for a support crew to provide water, food, changes of clothing, and first aid for blisters. All the serious contestants had handlers. When Lizzy reached 75 miles, Doug Reeves, who was at the race as a spectator and photographer, volunteered to become Lizzy's handler, so she could concentrate on the walking and thereby finish.

Lizzy did finish. In fact the nineteen-year-old athlete set a junior record for 100 miles. Her time of 23:50 was ten minutes better than she needed to become a Flatlander. She was the third woman to ever racewalk 100 miles in under twenty-four hours.

Lizzy has since set other records. Admittedly, there are relatively few female long-distance racewalkers, so a few of her records are earned by default. For instance, she was the first female to ever complete a two-day racewalk, so her distance of 140.25 miles was automatically the record for that forty-eight-hour race. On the other hand, many women racewalk marathons, so Lizzy's time of 4:25, in the 1985 Long Beach Marathon, is a legitimate U.S. racewalking record for females. Lizzy also holds the U.S. record for the 50-mile distance, with a time of 10:19. In the trials for the 1984 Los Angeles Olympics Lizzy Kemp came in seventh for the 10-kilometer racewalk.

It's clear that self-propelled endurance athletes are a mixed lot. Penny Dean, T. J. Key, Dale Sutton, and Lizzy Kemp are different from one another. But one characteristic they have in common is their tendency to seek increasingly greater challenges. Most of us walk or run or swim at some time or another, but why do a few of us do that to extremes and become endurance athletes?

Dale Sutton speculates that endurance athletics may be an inevitable by-product of basic human nature. He says, "It's a natural progression of activities. As an infant you had to start out crawling, then you went to walking. The natural progression for humans is to do more. We're trying to find out where the absolute maximum is. We don't know where it is. We haven't been stretched far enough to find out if you can run 1,000 miles nonstop. So the reason we run is it's natural. Some people are stronger than others, and those who are capable of doing these ultras, do them."

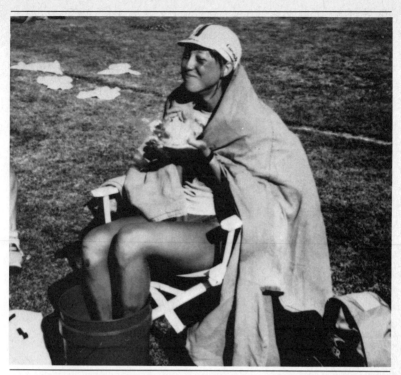

Lizzie Kemp takes a break during her record-breaking 48-hour racewalk.   PHOTO BY SIGNÉ ANN KEMP

Adriane Hughes paces Lizzy Kemp during the 48-hour racewalk.   PHOTO BY SIGNÉ ANN KEMP

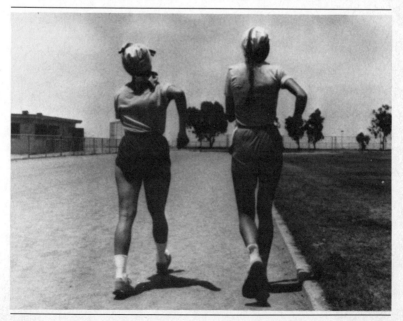

THE HUMAN ENGINES

*I*N A MANNER of speaking, cross-country skiers, rowers, and cyclists are the power plants for primitive transportation machines. Their muscle power makes their equipment move. In this chapter two "human engines" are profiled: John Howard, a professional cyclist, and Carol Duffy, an amateur Nordic skier.

IRONMAN HOWARD

"Boy, you're in deep doo-doo," barked the raspy-voiced army sergeant over the telephone. "The lieutenant colonel wants to talk to you. Hold on!"

John's benefactor at the Pentagon came on the line: "Young man, are you aware that you've been AWOL for the last month and a half? You have exactly thirty-six hours to report for duty at Fort Polk, Louisiana. Now get your ass in gear, and don't let me hear that you didn't get there on time."

John wasn't exactly a deserter, it's just that shortly after he won the gold medal at the Pan Am Games, the army had disbanded its improbable little unit of competitive cyclists. John didn't quite know what to do or where to go, so he took two weeks' leave and went home to wait for new orders at his folks' place in Springfield, Missouri. When the two weeks were up, and his new orders hadn't arrived, John just figured he'd stay there and wait some more. He watched the mailbox for a couple more weeks and no orders arrived. Pretty soon he had been home a month, and then that stretched into two months. Still no orders had come, but John's gnawing anxiety about his absence by then had turned into full-blown nightmares. In his dreams two plainclothed FBI agents, accompanied by a sadistic-looking MP, came to the door of his parents' house. Without comment, the MP shackled him and led him away to a horrible future within the walls of the federal penitentiary at Fort Leavenworth, Kansas.

John's apparent troubles with the army came at the end of one of the most successful years in his long career as a competitive cyclist. During that year, 1972, John had won the National Road Race Championship and the gold medal in the Pan Am Games. That year's successes were the culmination of a process that had begun when John watched the telecast of American Jack Simes cycling in the track events of the 1964 Olympics.

John, at six foot two, appears to carry virtually no fat. In fact, at one point his body fat was measured as low as 4 percent. He has very little upper body musculature compared to the watermelon-size quadriceps that power his legs. His neck and shoulders are rounded forward in a manner that gives him the ideal aerodynamic profile for a cyclist.

Now a thirty-eight-year-old pro rider, John has been a cyclist most of his life. One of the earliest photos that exists of John shows him astride a toy tractor. The toy tractor was pedal-driven. The bicycle was his basic mode of transportation throughout his grade school and high school years in Springfield, Missouri. He used to ride along with his friend George, Springfield's Western Union messenger. They would deliver the messages in record time so they could spend the rest of George's work hours riding in the countryside.

Meanwhile, John and his younger brother, Harry David—or H.D., as he was called—were both milers on the high school track team. John says, "Harry was always the better athlete. That used to embarrass me and make me jealous, because of normal sibling rivalry. He was a year younger and four seconds faster than me in the mile." But in his senior year John vindicated himself at the Ozark Conference Championships; he won his event, running the best mile of his track career, about a 4:40.

It was about a year before the Ozark meet that John had seen the Olympic cycling on television, and soon he had bought his first ten-speed bicycle (a Schwinn Continental, about the only ten-speed then available in the Midwest). He had thrown himself into the new sport. At John's urging, H.D. also tried cycling, but he didn't have the same enthusiasm for it as his older brother. "At the time I got interested in cycling, he got interested in girls," John explains.

John's early career as a cyclist began with noncompetitive American Youth Hostels (AYH) tours. He soon outdistanced the slow tourists and began looking around for something more competitive than the AYH rides. He wanted to race. At nineteen years old, he entered his first competition, a 105-mile road race from Oletha to Council Grove, Kansas.

That event was sanctioned by the United States Cycling Federation, but John says that in 1966 the officiation of midwestern competitive cycling was still pretty bush league. Another cyclist and John broke away from the small pack relatively early in the race. Unfortunately, that cyclist's father was the official referee, and John believes that nepotism prevented him from winning his very first race. When the pair got to Council Grove, the town where the race was to end, there was no formal finish line. The referee was supposed to drive ahead to Council Grove and record the results of the race. As John and the other cyclist rode through town, suddenly his companion pulled ahead. Just then, the other rider's father jumped from a car, waved a checkered flag and declared his son the winner.

Three months later both riders were in a criterium (repeated laps around a short course), the Tour of Springfield. John and his erstwhile drafting partner had broken from the pack again, but this time John didn't work with him. John simply rode away from him, leaving him in the dust as he went on to win the event.

John didn't do so well in his next major race, the Tour of Florrisant (a suburb of St. Louis). That tour was a criterium consisting of fifty laps around a 1-mile course. John was doing fine, staying up with the leaders, but the *pelotin* (pack) was both numerous and crammed onto a narrow road. Other riders had boxed him in. "During the maneuvering at close quarters," he recounts, "I couldn't deal with the traffic. Somebody crowded me in a turn. I went off the road, hit a culvert, tore up my front wheel and I crashed."

That's how John began collecting scars that make his knees look like relief maps of the Himalayas. But then, as now, his biggest concern was race performance: "I had my first shot at national-caliber competition, and I blew it."

It wasn't to be his last big-time race. He recalls, "It was at the end of the year [1966], in October, that I made my first real statement about who I was in the sport." He competed in the Wachter Memorial Race in St. Louis and finished fourth. The race was won by Eddie Doerr, who was then a seasoned champion in his mid-twenties. At the awards ceremony Doerr announced that young Howard, who had stayed right up with the big boys in the lead break, was one of the strongest candidates in the Midwest for the U.S. Olympic squad. That statement opened an undreamed-of vista for John. Traditionally, the membership of the U.S. Olympic Cycling Team had been drawn exclusively from the East Coast and West Coast riders.

Inspired by Doerr's remark, John redoubled his training. He increased his weekly distance and put in regular speed workouts. Bicycling became his most important and time-consuming activity. To support himself, he worked as a lifeguard. He and his brother also started a small woodcutting business. "We had a big old Ford flatbed truck, on which we could pile about two cords of firewood," he recounts. With chainsaws, splitting malls, and axes John and H.D. cut and prepared white oak for the fireplaces of Springfield and nearby communities. John fondly reminisces about the venture, "We got to the point where we could cut, split, and stack a cord of wood in an hour; I would do most of the main cutting, H.D. would do most of the lifting and stacking. We were fast." By living frugally at his parents' house, John could subsist on the lifeguarding and firewood business and have plenty of time left over to put in long hours training on the bicycle.

The workouts paid off, too. As a virtual unknown, he went to the trials for the 1968 Olympics in Agoura, California. Agoura, which since then has been engulfed by the Los Angeles megalopolis, was still rural in those days. "Out there on the country roads of Agoura," John says, "I surprised a lot of people; I came in second. They were asking, 'Who is this guy?' " He wasn't supposed to do so well. In essence the Olympic squad had already been selected, and this qualification race was to be just a formality to confirm the choices. When John went on that year to take the first of seven U.S. National Championships that he would ultimately win, it became clear that his victory in Agoura was not just a fluke. He made the team, although John recalls, "The coach told me afterward, 'You're the only person on the team I hadn't picked.' "

American cyclists have not always done as well at the Olympics as they did in 1984. In fact, between 1912 and 1984, not one Olympic cycling medal went to an American. The 1968 Olympics in Mexico City was no exception. At those Games John was the only American to even complete the road race, though he only placed among the top forty riders. John made the Olympic team twice more (1972 and 1976) and was eventually able to bring his road race finish up to thirteenth place at the Munich Olympics in 1972. At Mexico City in 1968, John also competed in the 100-kilometer team time trial. John's inexperience made the coaches reluctant to put him on the time trial team, but he turned out to be the strongest member.

That time trial did not pass without incident. John wrote an article for the July 1984 issue of *Bicycle Sport,* in which he reported, "I am pumping my bicycle tires for the 100 kilometer team time trial. A Mexican man, standing a scant five feet from me, raises a large-caliber pistol to his head, pulls the trigger and spatters his brains all over the sidewalk, my bicycle and my clean, lily-white American team jersey. Possibly a political activist, the suicide victim was wanted by the government and wished to make his death a spectacle." Four years later, at the Munich Olympics, John was only 100 feet away when Black September terrorists attacked the Israeli Olympic team.

When he returned from his first Olympics John wasn't sure what he wanted to do professionally. He was not too keen on resuming the firewood business, since H.D. had moved on to other activities. For the moment he lived on savings, competed full-time as an amateur, and enrolled in a few courses at a local university. But he had no firm occupational plans. Then in 1970 the local draft board solved his quandary for him. The Vietnam War was in full swing, and John looked like prime cannon fodder. Before he could blink an eye he had completed basic training.

John was an Olympic athlete, and he had heard that the army had Special Services units comprised of jocks who represented America in international competitions. Al Toefield, then the president of the United States Cycling Federation, knew a major at the Pentagon who was nominally in charge of such things. (The major, later promoted to lieutenant colonel, was the officer who would remind John that he was AWOL.) Toefield helped John apply for a transfer, but army paper often moves even slower than the soldiers themselves. Before any action could be taken on John's request, he was sent with his basic-training company to Advanced Infantry Training at Fort Polk, Louisiana. Very soon John was learning how to handle combat weapons, and he appeared to be on a fast track to the rice paddies of Vietnam.

At Fort Polk, John first went to his company commander to ask for help in getting his transfer untangled from the Pentagon web. The company commander was not receptive. Then John's company attended an orientation given by the captain's superior officer, a full-bird colonel in command of the battalion. In his welcoming remarks, the colonel said, "If any of you have any problems—personal or otherwise—you can jump the chain of command and come directly to see me. I'd welcome that."

John tells how he took the colonel's words at face value: "When we finished the orientation all the other troops went back to the barracks. I turned around and went straight to the colonel's office and met him there; I was waiting for him when he came back." John was in store for a great stroke of luck—the colonel was himself a competitive cyclist. The colonel had represented his college fraternity in the Little Indy 500, the race in Bloomington, Indiana, portrayed in the movie *Breaking Away*.

The colonel also knew how to cut red tape. He immediately gave John a three-day pass to go home and pick up his car and cycling equipment. Allowing soldiers in Advanced Infantry Training to have a car on base was virtually unheard of, but the colonel solved that problem by excusing John from the remainder of the combat training. Besides, he would need the car for transportation to bike races, and the colonel wanted to do everything he could to make the Olympic cyclist comfortable. John's only problem at that point was that he didn't own a car, but he quickly solved that dilemma himself by buying a shiny new Volkswagen bug.

With the colonel making inquiries on his behalf, it wasn't long before John had orders to a special detachment of competitive cyclists that was stationed at Fort Wadsworth, in Staten Island, New York (where the New York City Marathon now starts). When John got to New York he found himself in the company of some of the finest cyclists in the country, riders who had either enlisted or been drafted and had been assembled at Fort Wadsworth from all the military services. Some of the top American riders of the day were there: Dave Chauner, Steve Woznick, Mike Hiltner, Bill Guazo, Larry Swantner, and Cliff Halsey.

Two or three days a week the bicycle platoon and its bicycles were loaded on an army truck and driven out to Long Island. There the military cyclists hammered the beautiful country roads and hills from Oyster Bay to Montauk Point. On alternate days they took a five-cent ferry ride from Staten Island to Manhattan, and they trained on the loop in Central Park. They trained hard, partly because they knew that to be cut from the team meant an almost certain ticket to Vietnam. "But I wanted to train," John says. "For the first time ever I had been paid to ride my bike, and it was perfect for me." John decided to make the best of a good situation; he painted his fine Eisentrout racing bicycle olive-drab (army green) and put decals on it that said TEAM ARMY. He tried to convince his teammates to paint their bikes in army colors, too, but John says, "The others wouldn't do that; it just wasn't their style."

The army sent its team of cyclists to amateur competitions in Europe, the United States, and South America. The riders, ostensibly competing as individuals, did well, too. After the 1972 Pan Am Games, most of the riders were due to leave the army fairly soon, so the bicycling unit was disbanded. John was due out in only a few months when he had taken his "unauthorized" leave. When the lieutenant colonel's call abruptly returned him to army life, John wasn't sure what punishment awaited him at Fort Polk. Upon arrival there, he was saved by the inefficiency and inconsistencies of huge bureaucracies. "They hadn't been informed of any of this," John says, "and they treated me like I was a hero." A month or so later John left the army.

Over the next seven years John was employed by various bicycle manufacturers as an athlete and public relations manager. He was a successful competitor, but by 1979 he was ready for a change. He recalls, "I read the *Sports Illustrated* article about the Ironman. Like a lot of people, I was impressed by the race. I found it hard to believe, but at the same time I realized that I could do well in that event."

John went to Oahu in February 1980 with the intention of winning the Ironman Triathlon. Unfortunately, he was humbled by the strong surf at Waikiki. During the 2.4-mile swim he swallowed a great deal of saltwater. After his swamping, the champion cyclist was able to make up lost time on the 112-mile bike ride around Oahu. Distance running, which he had only begun a few months earlier, was not his strength. His marathon time was much slower than he wanted. He finished the triathlon in third place, behind Dave Scott and Chuck Newmann.

Most people would be ecstatic to finish third at the Ironman, but John felt he was capable of much more. The event had been won by Dave Scott, a true triathlete. Scott's training put equal emphasis on all three sports. John recognized that his own strategy had been to win the event by virtue of overwhelming superiority on the bicycle. He vowed to do his multisport homework in order to win next year's race. John became a devotee and advocate of well-rounded cross-training. He reasoned that triathletes can be truly fit because the whole effect of their training is greater than the parts.

On Valentine's Day 1981 John was in Kona, Hawaii, competing in the first Ironman to be staged at that new location. He finished the event in a time of 9:38.29, winning it by a substantial margin. The bicyclist had become a triathlete.

For the next few years, John continued to compete in bike races and triathlons as a professional. During that period he earned his living from race prizes and sponsorships.

In 1982, John rode against Lon Haldeman, Michael Shermer, and John Marino in the Great American Bike Race (GABR), predecessor of the transcontinental event now called the Race Across AMerica. He made it across the country in about ten days, finishing second to Haldeman. The effort nearly wiped him out. After crossing the southwestern desert he almost withdrew from the race, a victim of heat exhaustion. Instead, he slept for over five hours and resumed the race. While he was asleep he slipped into last place, but he caught and passed Shermer and Marino the following days.

Almost a year after the GABR John pushed himself again to overcome an endurance challenge. On Memorial Day 1983, he rode in the Pepsi Challenge 24-Hour Bicycle Marathon in New York City. The race consisted of twenty-four hours of laps around Central Park, with the victory going to the rider who completed the most miles. John did an honest day's work, covering a greater distance than any of the other riders despite eighteen miserable hours of rain. He cycled 514 miles, a new American record for twenty-four hours.

It appears as though John's competitive swan song may be a fast event rather than an endurance event. On July 20, 1985, he achieved an unusual record, one he had stalked for the previous four years. At this writing—and perhaps for a long time to come—John holds the bicycle land-speed record.

If you don't know how fast that is, before reading further, guess the speed. Keep in mind that this is a "motor-pacing" record. That is, the cyclist pedals in the slipstream of a fast motor vehicle. If you guessed anything under 60 miles per hour, then revise upward. Way back in 1898 Charles N. Murphy set the first bicycle land-speed record while riding behind a Long Island Railroad train on a stretch of specially smoothed track. He earned the nickname "Mile-a-Minute Murphy" by bicycling a mile at the remarkable speed of 63 miles per hour. Murphy was very nearly killed when the engineer slowed the train too soon, but his alert handlers managed to pull him aboard without injury. Bicycle land-speed records are tests of courage and skill, as well as feats of strength.

During the eighty-eight years after Murphy set his record there were two world wars, the airplane and atom bomb were invented, and a man walked on the moon. You might imagine that Murphy's mark has been vastly improved upon. It has. Motorpacers no longer bicycle behind trains; they now use race cars.

When John sought his record, he rode behind Rick Vesco's Bonneville Streamliner. Like Allan Abbott, the Los Angeles physician and motorcycle racer who held the record (138.674 miles per hour) before him, John rode on the hard-packed, dead-level Bonneville Salt Flats in Utah. The Salt Flats are the bottom of a dried-up, prehistoric lake. That desert is often used for ultra-high-speed record setting because vehicles can drive, skid, or careen for many miles without hitting a bump or any other obstruction.

So how fast did John go? When he finally set his record, John went 152.28 miles per hour.

What will he do for an encore? Well, it seems that the land-speed record is a pretty tough act to follow. There's no telling what he may try next, but for the most part, John seems to compete a lot less than before. Maybe after more than twenty years as a bike racer he figures he should make a living from his sport while he still can. He has started a company that sells bicycles and cycling clothing at the high and medium levels of the price scale. John also writes books and articles about bicycling and fitness and lectures on those topics.

His present role in athletics seems to be that of a player-coach. He teaches training methods, but he hasn't completely abandoned competition. His own training is still a daily activity, but now it is more for fun and maintenance of health than for improvement as a com-

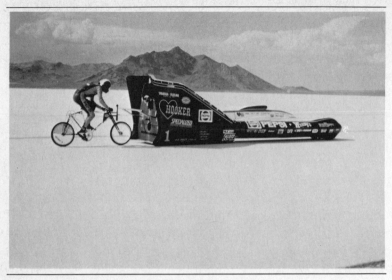

John Howard at 152.28 miles per hour.

John Howard at 28 miles per hour.

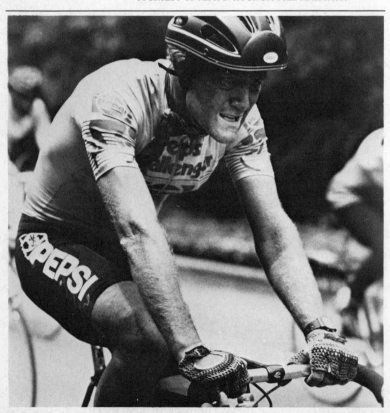

petitor. John says he plans to continue his daily workouts as long as he lives. He will probably always be a threat in age-group competition.

CAROL DUFFY

There once was a lady who lived in a shoe, she had so many children she didn't know what to do. So she became a cross-country skier.

Carol Duffy has eleven children and six grandchildren. She has demonstrated other forms of endurance as well. In 1980 Carol and her husband, Tom, became the first two skiers to complete their Worldloppet Passports by skiing all nine of the grueling cross-country events that then constituted the Worldloppet series. (The shortest of those events was 42 kilometers, the longest was 89 kilometers, and one of them, the 55-kilometer Birkebeiner-Rennet, in Norway, required that the Duffys ski with 12-pound packs on their backs.) Two years after they traveled the globe to do Worldloppet, Carol and Tom tackled the entire American Classic Series in just one year's time. The Classic Series includes the Tour of Raddison Bike Race (217 miles), the Muskelunge Lake Swim (2.6 miles), the Log-Driver Marathon footrace (26.2 miles), the Leif Erikson Roller-Ski event (26.2 miles), and the Birkebeiner Nordic Ski Race (34.1 miles).

Carol was born into a family of five children. She was the only female in that brood. Two of her brothers were older than she and two were younger. Her brothers were continuously engaged in sports, always lifting weights or playing football. One of her siblings, Ken Yackel, was a hockey player on the U.S. Olympic Team in the 1952 Winter Games at Oslo, Norway. Ken went on to play hockey as a professional for the Boston Bruins.

Carol emulated her athletic brothers. She recalls, "I liked sports. I always wanted to do what they wanted to do; I didn't play with dolls, that's for sure."

Carol and Tom married in 1955, and by 1971 she had given birth to ten children, four girls and six boys. Understandably, the rigors of motherhood cut into the time that Carol had for purely selfish activity, but she recalls, "Through those years, whenever I was able to do something for myself, it always had something to do with athletics." Sports come easily to Carol.

She and her husband Tom lived in Hayward, Wisconsin, a small town close to the Telemark Ski Resort which Tony Wise was then developing into a cross-country center. When Carol was introduced to Nordic skiing, about two years before she gave birth to her eleventh child, the new sport clicked for her immediately. Carol had taken a cross-country skiing lesson from Eric Errson, a Norwegian instructor at Telemark who barely spoke English. Somehow Errson managed to tell her how to get aboard the skis. Carol describes her experience: "When I put those skis on for the first time it was such a wonderful, marvelous feeling."

It wasn't long before Errson had told Carol about a ski race that Tony Wise would soon promote. That was the very first American Birkebeiner, in February 1973. Carol thought, "My God, I've only been on these skis about five or ten times; how can I enter a race?" Despite her initial fears, she entered the 29-kilometer Korteloppet, or short race, that accompanied the Birkie. To her surprise she won the event.

That success changed Carol's life: "You don't ever get medals for having babies and changing diapers, and it's so much harder work. I was used to doing things when I was tired. Maybe I was up all night with a baby, but I still got up at six o'clock, made breakfast, got the rest of the kids off to school, and kept going, going, going. Here I had just had this wonderful fun and I got a medal, and I won a prize. I thought, 'Gee, I like the way this feels. I'll do it again, and maybe I'll win another prize.' " She entered many other races. Along the way she picked up numerous age-group and women's division prizes.

Carol Duffy is an unlikely candidate to be the first person to complete the entire Worldloppet Series. The responsibility for eleven children is not generally conducive to international travel and full-bore endurance training. According to Carol, many people told her and Tom that they wouldn't be able to do it. In fact, their original intention had been to do just two of the races. But that winter two of the Duffys' older daughters were home from college and willing to mind the younger children. At the same time, Tom Duffy was able to take some time off from his law practice. The previous summer the Duffys had trained by roller-skiing or running each morning between 5:30 and 7:00 A.M. To build their upper-body strength for poling, they had rowed also. Everything had fallen into place. Traveling to compete in Worldloppet was logistically possible, and they were in good condition for endurance sport. In just two months' time Carol and Tom skied in seven cross-country races, six of them in different European countries. The next winter they skied in two more of the races to complete the series.

In one of the Worldloppet races, the 1979 River Rouge in Canada, Carol was the first woman over thirty to finish and the third woman overall. Not bad work for your average forty-four-year-old mother of eleven.

The Great American Classic Series posed a different sort of problem for Carol. No European travel was involved. Not only are all the events local, but they also are spread across the year, so you can train

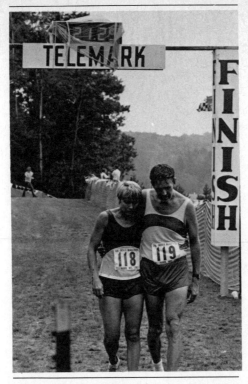

Carol and Tom Duffy at the first Log Driver Marathon.

COURTESY OF TERRELL BOETTCHER

for each one in its turn. Moreover, the sequence of the events—bicycling, roller-skiing, running, and swimming in the summer, and the Birkie in the winter—provided the ideal cross-training for a Nordic skier. But Carol had two major obstacles to overcome: she had never done much bicycling and she was deathly afraid of swimming.

The bicycle problem was solved in a relatively straightforward manner. She and Tom got on the roads and bicycled a lot. They built their mileage, and they both were able to finish the two-day 217-mile Tour of Raddison. The fear of swimming defied such an easy solution.

"From the time I was a little girl," Carol explains, "I had bad experiences with people dunking me. I'm terrified of the water." Besides, the Muskelunge Swim is in a cold-water lake full of creepy, crawly animals and plants. Carol describes her reaction to weeds in the water as one of absolute paranoia. When she began to train for the Muskelunge Swim all she could manage was a doggie paddle and a pathetic sidestroke. How would she complete the 2.6-mile lake swim if she was incapable of swimming the length of a pool and was petrified of drowning?

First she desensitized herself by swimming in a relatively warm and safe pool. During the early-morning hours and weekends Carol trained in the small swimming pool at the Telemark Lodge. The Telemark pool had not really been designed for lap swimming; it was more suitable for poolside socializing. But it was the best pool she could get, and Wisconsin lakes and rivers are too cold for much swimming until late in the summer. The race was scheduled for the Fourth of July. Still, she persevered, building her muscles for swimming.

Finally, two weeks before the event, the water at nearby Namekagon River was warm enough to permit Carol to do a trial swim. She describes how that swim in the river affected her confidence: "I thought I could do it then, but that didn't take away the fear." But she took sensible steps to deal with that problem, too.

Carol enlisted the support of a personal lifeguard, Carolin Kampman, an eighteen-year-old German exchange student who was then staying at the Duffy household. Kampman is an excellent swimmer, and Carol offered to pay her entry fee in the race if she would swim alongside as extra protection.

The water was a comfortable 70 degrees on race day, and Carol swam the backstroke and sidestroke. With a tone of fright still lingering in her voice, Carol recalls, "I was so proud of myself. I swam through the weeds without getting hysterical."

Endurance sport often means much more to people than just an opportunity to exercise. Take Carol Duffy's Muskelunge Swim: "I really am sincere when I say I am afraid of the water. When I finished that swim, I felt that I had overcome fears that had been with me for forty years. That was more important than how long it took me or what time I came in. I really conquered something inside of myself."

Carol still hasn't acquired the same love of the water as she says her husband has. Nor have the nonbicycling Duffys become avid cyclists. Nonetheless, the special lure of endurance challenges has broadened Carol. That first Birkebeiner in 1973 has led her to overcome fears and experience sports she might otherwise never have attempted.

Initially, it took strength of purpose for Carol to become so deeply involved in endurance sport. During the early 1970s Carol remembers, "We wouldn't think of putting on our running clothes and running out the front door and down the street." The small community of Hayward would have been aghast at such outlandish behavior. Yet the Duffys resisted the pressure to conform, and in retrospect Carol is certain that her health has been a major beneficiary. Now the neighbors who once ridiculed her are out walking or jogging themselves.

Carol was thirty-eight when she first skied the Birkie and discovered endurance athletics. Before that, her social life included a lot of eating and drinking. She says, "If my children were doing what I did at age thirty-five, had that kind of a life-style, I wouldn't like it. If my children choose the life-style I have now, I would be very proud of them."

Modeling a fitness life-style has worked. The Duffy children are athletes. Carol has run marathons with one of her daughters and two of her sons. Some of her children compete in log-rolling, a classic lumberjack sport that requires both skill and cardiovascular fitness. Some of her children also ice-skate and play hockey like their uncle Ken.

Two citizen athletes with eleven children need exceptional drive to pursue endurance sport as enthusiastically as the Duffys. Carol says, "We were so motivated, I wish I could get that same motivation back." Carol feels as though she is in a bit of an athletic slump now. She still runs in the summer and will continue to ski the Birkie, but she lacks the specific challenge that motivated her to do Worldloppet and the Classic Series. She wants to do something different, and she probably will, when she decides what it is. Next summer, she does plan to join a half dozen other women on an all-female canoeing expedition on Alaskan rivers.

At fifty-one, what does this endurance athlete plan for her twilight years, twenty or thirty years hence? She says, "I want to go out and just have a log cabin with no running water, and no indoor toilet, and make it very difficult to survive. I want to be one of those eccentric old ladies who grows her own herbs and rides her bicycle into town. Once our last one has graduated, that's what I'm thinking about. Or who knows, maybe I'll join the Peace Corps."

THE MULTIATHLETES

*T*O UNDERSTAND A new sport you must know what makes the athletes tick. First, consider Dale Basescu, a professional triathlete who is almost up there with the big boys—Dave Scott, Scott Molina, Scott Tinley, and Mark Allen. As they used to say in the rental car business, "Dale tries harder." He has to; the triathlon is his career. Then look at a group portrait of two female professional triathletes, Jacqueline Shaw and Colleen Cannon, who went pro because that's the best way they know to enjoy a playful, fulfilling life of adventure and travel.

DALE BASESCU

Ring, ring, click—then a recording cuts in. A voice reminiscent of Peter Sellers, mimicking the accent of a Hindu holy man, comes over the phone line:

> This is the Ipson Halcyon Guru Answering Service for Dale Basescu. Dale has just returned from his sojourn to the high peaks of the Colorado Rockies, where he was not only humbled by the majesty and the beauty, but by the high altitude and his crumby eighth-place finish in the Denver Triathlon. Dale can't come to the phone right now, he is out on his bike doing penance for his worst race of the season. But, upon his return, I will deliver your message to him personally. And don't forget the inspirational words of our great master: "He who has many weeds in his garden should eat a pepperoni pizza."

During triathlon season, Dale Basescu's callers are very likely to get a recorded message. He is either out training or he is on the road—competing. Dale is one of a few dozen professionals who stand apart from the 1.1 million amateur triathletes.

Dale is not living in opulence. His modest apartment in Encinitas, California, has been furnished sparsely in early garage sale style. Dale explains, "I have to be a master of budgeting to do what I'm doing. I put away more money than people making a lot more than I do." Yet, judging from the various "trick" bicycles that hang from the

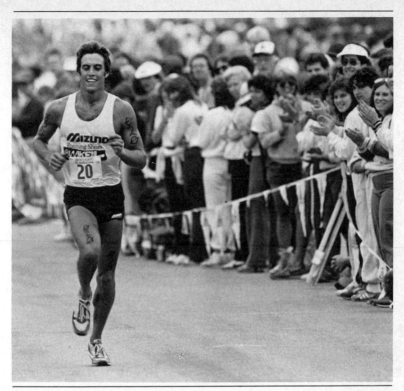

Dale Basescu enjoying a victory. COURTESY OF BUD LIGHT USTS

kitchen ceiling or lean against the Spartan furniture, it is clear that Basescu is not miserly. Those racing machines definitely were not bought from Manny, Moe, and Jack down at the local Pep Boys. Dale has merely opted to follow a professional sport for which the financial rewards still have not developed fully.

Dale apologetically explains the apparent extravagance in the bicycle department: "I need a new bike every season. They get all torqued out. You stress them a lot. The lugs loosen, and they're no longer responsive. Ideally, I should have two good bikes; one for training and one for competing." The bicycles are tools of his trade.

Dale, twenty-nine years old, was born in New York City, but left there as a small child and grew up in Boulder, Colorado. He attended the University of Arizona and graduated from Colorado State University. He swam intercollegiately on an athletic scholarship and was ranked thirty-eighth in the world for the 400-meter individual medley. For the 200-meter individual medley he was ranked twenty-fourth nationally.

Dale majored in communications, and his ambition was to be an entertainer. Dale sings, plays the piano and guitar, and writes music, including a few recent ballads about triathlons. He has acted and worked professionally as a musician.

When he graduated college in 1979, Dale lived for a while in his van—a large vehicle that could accommodate the spinet piano that he hauled around with him everywhere. He didn't quite know where else to go, so he headed for Nashville, Tennessee. The country-and-western mecca seems an odd choice for Basescu. His preferred styles are soft rock and folk. He's flexible, though, and will sing whatever is appropriate for the band with which he is working.

In Tennessee, Dale got some small acting jobs, performed music at clubs and restaurants, and worked other pick-up jobs outside of show biz as necessary. During this period he continued his fitness activities and was mildly interested when he read the *Sports Illustrated* feature about Tom Warren's victory in the 1979 Ironman. He was struggling to make it as a songwriter, so when he heard about the Nashville Triathlon—a 1.5-mile swim, 50-mile bike ride, and 13.1-mile run—he took a bold step. He launched a campaign to get a sponsor for the event.

Dale's athletic résumé caught the eye of Fred Dettwiller, the Nashville distributor of Miller Lite, and suddenly he was a sponsored, professional jock. Not megabucks, just enough to help buy a good bike and running shoes. He trained for about two weeks. Perhaps Dale's cardiovascular base from swimming pulled him through, or perhaps an "I can lick the world" attitude compensated for his inadequate training. "I had a swimmer's upper body, and these spindly little legs," Dale recalls. Surprisingly, he won the Nashville event, and not by a squeaker either. He broke the previous course record by forty-five minutes and beat all the other entrants by thirty-five minutes.

"I had no limitations mentally, because it was the first time I did it," Dale explains. "But physically I did have limitations." Later, he believes the opposite occurs: training and honing expand athletes' physical limits, but then their awareness of the potential pain puts many mental limitations on performance. After his first triathlon Dale felt intense pain, particularly in his legs, but in all other parts of his body as well. The soft tissues in his legs and his knees hurt. His Achilles tendons were swollen. He says, "I pushed myself beyond my physical limitations, because as far as I was concerned I had no limitations." During the event he had suppressed the immediate pain and surrendered completely to the exhilaration of swimming, biking, and running.

There was no prize money at the Nashville Triathlon—his sponsorship had been limited to equipment—but still he had discovered that it was possible to get some money for having fun. He was hooked on professional athletics. Meanwhile, the publicity did some good for his entertainment career. WSM-TV in Tennessee sporadically asked him to appear as a fitness commentator.

He had a toehold on a career in regional broadcasting, but he was not at home in the Southeast. The culture and way of life were alien to him, so he gave in to the old wanderlust. He threw his piano back in the van, packed up, and headed for Florida. There he played piano bars for a living and learned everything he could about physical fitness and exercise physiology. The stimulation of his new sports— bicycling and running—nicely compensated for the boredom that he had begun to feel when he swam.

He now served two masters: amateur athletics and show biz. When he sold the old spinet in Florida, it looked as though the balance was beginning to tip in favor of an athletic career. But he had always regarded his modest triathlon sponsorship in Nashville as a fluke. In 1980 there was no professional triathlon circuit. He hardly gave professional sport a second thought when he moved to Los Angeles. He took an apartment in Santa Monica and gave up the vagabond existence of the van resident. Dale threw himself into the life of endless auditions and semipro acting in Equity-waiver theater.

It's called "Equity-waiver" because it's technically nonunion amateur acting, which doesn't require a membership in Actors Equity. Building a reputation for your skill as an Equity-waiver actor is one of the few ways to break through the catch-22 of the Hollywood star machine: you can't get an acting job unless you have a union card, and you can't get a union card unless you already have an acting job. Hence, Equity-waiver theater in Los Angeles is often first-rate and the competition for amateur roles is keen.

Dale was surviving on the hopes and promises of a town where, he says, "You have to scam for anything you get." He was getting himself coffeehouse gigs as a guitar vocalist, he was doing well in non-Equity acting roles, and ultimately he even got a competent theatrical agent. At one point he was being considered for a coveted role in "Days of Our Lives." It is easy to see why: Dale has precisely the sort of polished good looks that one would associate with a soap opera star. But that's as close as Dale has gotten to national, daytime TV.

"If I had gotten the soap opera part, that would have taken me down a different road," Dale speculates. "During all this," he says, "I always kept in fairly good shape." He had been swimming on the Santa Monica Masters Swim Team, and gradually Dale's training began to take up a larger proportion of his time than auditioning for roles.

While in Los Angeles, he finished in second place at the Castaic Lake Triathlon—a 1,000-yard swim, 18-mile bike ride, and 10-kilometer run—and remembers feeling "euphoric" because of it. He was unsponsored and there were no cash prizes at Castaic Lake, but at the time he felt, "To get money for something like that would be incredible, because it's just pure enjoyment."

Dale met and befriended Harald Johnson, a fellow masters swim-

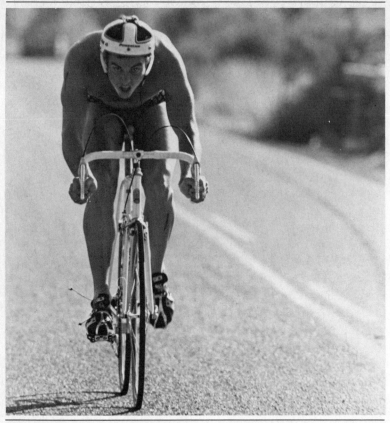

Dale Basescu hammering.

mer, who was then art director of *Swim-Swim* magazine, which served the needs of the small community of endurance swimmers. (Unfortunately for its cult following, *Swim-Swim* is now defunct.) That was about the time *Swim-Swim*'s publisher, Michael Gilmore, was gearing up to produce the slick, full-color *Triathlon* magazine. Johnson ultimately moved over to the new magazine as editorial director.

Harald and Dale went to dinner together after one workout with the Santa Monica Masters Swim Club, and Harald casually told Dale about the U.S. Triathlon Series, which race promoter Jim Curl was just then starting up.

In retrospect, Dale recognizes that the dinner conversation was one of those casual-seeming discussions that turns a person's life completely around. Johnson told Basescu that the U.S. Triathlon Series would include prize money for the pros. Basescu recalls telling Johnson, "I don't even want to hear about that." He hastens to add, "But of course I did want to find out more."

Dale found out lots more. He became a professional triathlete, realizing along the way that he has a special talent for the so-called "sprint" events, such as the USTS races, which include 1.5 kilometers of swimming, 40 kilometers of bicycling, and 10 kilometers of running. (Of course, the sprints still require several hours to complete, so he merely has to work that much harder for a short period than he would in a longer endurance contest.)

Basescu now earns his living from a Nike sponsorship and prize money at races, and he has become savvy about those matters, too. When he started out he felt honored to work for a pair of running shoes and a free bicycle. Now he has costs for competition—such as international travel—and he makes sure that sponsors or promoters pick up those tabs. His sponsor also provides him with a modest monthly stipend. He's not yet at the point where he loses sleep over tax shelters. On the other hand, if he keeps winning races, as he has so far this season, he'll be able to continue making a living doing what he enjoys. As he puts it, "The triathlon keeps me in rice cakes and bananas."

He has moved to Encinitas, a small beach town north of San Diego, where it's much easier to train than in Los Angeles. It's also easier to keep track of what's going on in the sport there. Many of his competitors live in nearby communities. In his new home, he also has managed to continue his entertainment career in a low-key way: he plays guitar a few times a week at a local vegetarian restaurant.

One of the reasons Dale finds it easy to live frugally is that he doesn't have many entertainment costs. He says, "All I pay for is food and living, and my entertainment comes because I get to race and travel all over the world—free. What more entertainment is there than that?" Dale obviously enjoys his work. He explains, "What I do is entertaining, getting out on my bike and riding around and running. I wouldn't want to do anything else, except maybe play the guitar, and I do that too."

It's not all roses, though. There's pressure to perform. Sometimes the enthusiasm is not there for a race, and he says he can't consider doing an event for which there is no prospect of pay. There are only so many races his body can endure in one season, and he has to earn a living. Having to win has taken a little of the fun out of the triathlon. Often now he has to work so hard in training or in a race that the satisfaction only comes later when he congratulates himself for pushing through the pain.

And there are general dissatisfactions. He feels that the top four competitors in the sport—Dave Scott, Scott Molina, Scott Tinley, and Mark Allen—get the lion's share of media coverage. He perceives himself as just below the cutoff: number five. He's quick to add that the leaders deserve credit for their obvious strength, skill, and poise under pressure. He feels, however, that the media ought to help develop the identities of some of the other competitors so the fans will understand the depth of talent in this endurance sport, in which the first ten finishers are often separated by only a few seconds.

Then there's the drafting rule, his pet peeve. In the 1985 Los Angeles USTS race Basescu was way out front during the bicycle portion, when he was overtaken by a group of about ten competitors riding together despite the regulation against drafting. A pace line of bicyclists has a substantial aerodynamic advantage over a rider working by himself. It is estimated by scientists that drafting may be worth an extra mile per hour per rider—for up to about eight or nine riders in a pack. That's a big benefit. Those who ride in a pack go much faster and arrive at the bicycle finish with a lot more energy left for the run. Dale ended up in fifth place in that Los Angeles race and the drafting cyclists were not penalized.

Race officials generally justify the antidrafting rule on two grounds: drafting is dangerous for the majority of triathletes who, as novice racers, are inexperienced in bike handling at close quarters; and it is feared that elite triathletes would otherwise hire "domestiques" (servants) who swim and bicycle well and thus could pull their "masters" up to a lead position going into the run. Then the domestique would fade or drop out of the event altogether. That system, which is common in bicycle racing, might compromise the integrity of the triathlon. Perhaps it would, and perhaps it wouldn't, but one thing is clear: Basescu doesn't like the status quo.

What particularly irks Dale is that the drafters who passed him at the Los Angeles race weren't disqualified, whereas a year earlier, in the Atlanta USTS Triathlon, he was penalized ten minutes for the same offense. He lost cash when he was penalized at Atlanta, and at Los Angeles, because the other riders weren't disciplined, he finished almost out of the money. He considered his $200 prize for fifth place so unfair under the circumstances that he tore up the check in protest at the awards ceremony. But he doesn't blame the riders or even the officiation. He blames the rule. Since the rule has cut him in both directions, he sees it as an unavoidable and irrational double-bind. He believes that efforts to enforce it better are doomed to failure. According to Dale, the top triathletes are so close to each other in ability that grouping on the bike ride is inevitable. This is particularly the case if the road is narrow, as it was in Los Angeles. Dropping the rule is the only solution that would please Dale.

Despite the demands of the sport and his dissatisfaction with some of the rules and working conditions, Dale's attitude seems almost incurably positive. When he catches himself griping about the sport, he asks himself, "What would you like to do better right now?" Then he realizes that he really feels privileged to earn his rice cakes doing what other people consider play. Even the antidrafting rule ultimately inspires an optimistic response by Dale: it's incentive for him to radically improve his running in order to compensate for anything that happens during the bike ride. He now can run 10 kilometers in thirty-three minutes, and he wants to lower that to about thirty-one minutes.

Nearing thirty, Dale believes that we all peak at some age, but that age may be later than previously supposed. As evidence, he points to Olympic gold medalist Carlos Lopes—who at thirty-eight briefly held the marathon world record (2:07.11). He looks forward to a long athletic career. Still, he keeps his options open. Dale continues to write songs, and he believes that the notoriety he gains from the triathlon will certainly help him if he actively resumes his acting career. He still wants to break into television or movies.

Acting is a profession for which many are called but few are chosen. The odds are against Dale, but then again only one person out of hundreds can win a triathlon. Dale does what is necessary to achieve some of his ambitions. He scarcely trained for his first triathlon, but he trains ferociously now. Look for him soon, at a theater near you.

COLLEEN CANNON AND JACQUELINE SHAW

One could argue that Canadian triathlete Jacqueline Shaw is the recipient of the stiffest, most expensive traffic fine in history. Shaw competed in a 1984 event at Lake Tahoe that bills itself as the "world's toughest triathlon." With over 15,000 feet of cumulative vertical climb on the bike ride and a course slightly longer than that of the Ironman—2.5-mile swim, 120-mile bike, and 27-mile run—the Tahoe event's claim may well be valid. Only about half the participants finish. Jacqueline enjoyed the stunning scenery, and she was the first woman to finish. It looked like she was in the catbird seat; the prize for the first female finisher was $10,000. Not bad pay for a day's work in some of the most beautiful surroundings on the planet.

Then it was learned that out on the bicycle course she had left an intersection about five seconds before the light turned green. Understand, she had stopped her bicycle, but you know how it is at a red light when there's no traffic and you're in a hurry. Jacqueline, who had a comfortable thirty-five-minute margin over the second finisher, feels that it might have been fair to punish her by giving her a time penalty. Anything up to thirty-four minutes and fifty-nine seconds would have been acceptable to her.

Many triathlons require that bicyclists adhere to the traffic laws,

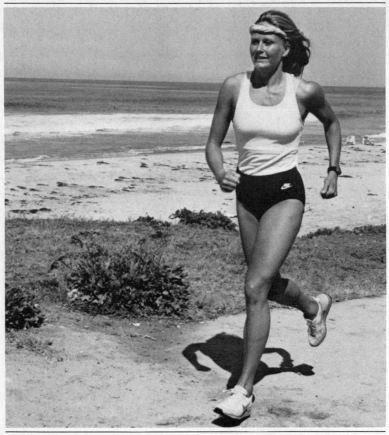

Jacqueline Shaw training at Del Mar, California.

PHOTO BY ALBERT GROSS

because the road is not closed for the event. Local authorities may have needed to be placated because some riders had flouted this event's strict rules on traffic signals. Possibly the race promoters had to make an example of somebody to save the event for future years. Although others had also run stoplights, nobody else got in trouble. Whatever the reason, Jacqueline was disqualified for running the red light and the prize money was given to the second female finisher.

It is characteristic of Jacqueline Shaw that she does not seem bitter about the decision. Some people might have fumed and fussed, others might have sued for the $10,000. But Jacqueline simply made plans to win the prize at next year's race.

Shaw's base of operations at the moment is southern California. If you needed to contact her during triathlon season you might have better luck looking for her in Oregon, Brazil, Australia, or Holland than in Del Mar, California, where she gets her mail. Although she is a resident alien in the United States, she will always retain her

Canadian citizenship. "I love my country," says the native of Calgary, Alberta.

Shaw, who is now twenty-nine years old, has been an athlete most of her life. As youngsters, she and her three older brothers took full advantage of the abundant outdoor activities near home. Calgary is on the eastern slope of the Canadian Rockies. From her earliest junior high school days, Jacqueline played on every team she could join: basketball, field hockey, gymnastics, track, swimming, and whatever else came up. At the University of Calgary, where she majored in mathematics and physical education, Shaw was forced to choose just one sport. She opted for basketball and was ranked at the top of the league. Shaw went on to play with the Canadian National team.

During college summers and later, when she was teaching mathematics and physical education, Shaw got involved in flat-water kayaking. She paddled all the way to the Nationals, but the 1,000-meter flat-water competitions weren't exciting enough for her. She graduated to white-water kayaking. Exhilarating shots down the rapids, in which she might cover five or six miles in just twenty minutes, were more to her liking. As she says, "We went down some real hairy stuff." She made it to the Nationals in white-water kayaking, too.

Jacqueline wants to be where the action is. Her enthusiasm and energy are contagious. Talk to her for just a few minutes and it becomes perfectly clear how this woman, who had a thirty-five-minute lead, could lose $10,000 because she didn't want to wait five more seconds at a traffic signal. Not that she is impulsive; she is just adventurous. Jacqueline is aware that she has followed her own instinct for adventure. "If I had taken my mom's advice I'd be back in Calgary married with two kids, I'm sure."

As much as she loves her homeland, there is no way that Calgary could have held Jacqueline Shaw. She would have exploded. Instead she indulged her thirst for adventure. She left her teaching duties behind her and traveled in Europe and the Middle East. She worked on a kibbutz in Israel, and she taught windsurfing and tended bar in Tahiti.

By some tangled, circuitous route she ended up in Los Angeles with a problem: "How do I get back home to Canada?" Most people would have solved that problem by buying a bus, train, or airline ticket. Naturally, Jacqueline bought a bicycle and equipped it with panniers to carry her personal effects. She bicycled 2,500 miles by herself, heading up the Pacific Coast from Los Angeles, turning right at Vancouver, and crossing the Rockies to reach Calgary.

She arrived home in May. "By summer," she says, "I got itchy again, so I went and cycled another 2,000 miles, around Montana and

Wyoming." Then Jacqueline saw the Ironman Triathlon on television, and that was about all it took to set her off. Since she is a Canadian, it was no problem gaining admission to the 1983 race. The qualification system reserves 25 percent of its starting positions for foreign applicants.

Meanwhile, an acquaintance suggested that she might become a pretty good bike racer. She attacked bicycle racing with the same élan she had shown for basketball and white-water kayaking. In July of 1983 she went to the Canadian Nationals in a fourth sport, bicycling. Although her cycling career had only included five races, Jacqueline came in fifth in the time trial event at the Nationals.

Clearly, Shaw is a versatile athlete. She was ripe for a multisport event such as the triathlon, but by August the Ironman was only a few months off, and Jacqueline still hadn't done any running or swimming. She could have buckled down to swimming and running, but she says, "To be a well-rounded person, I thought I should ride down the East Coast." Off she went on a 1,500-mile solo bicycle trek from Toronto to North Carolina.

At the end of August, with the Ironman just a little more than one month away, she drove to San Francisco. En route she commenced her running workouts. Her first training run was a 10-mile jaunt down into and back out of the Grand Canyon. She started at about 8,000 feet at the Canyon's south rim. On her way down the Kaibob Trail to the Canyon's floor at 4,000 feet, she got four blue toes. The descent was more painful than the ascent for the neophyte runner, who says, "I was never so glad to run up a hill in my life."

While on the West Coast she did one major training event, the Santa Barbara Triathlon, whose distances are half those of the Ironman. To Jacqueline's utter astonishment, she was the first woman finisher. Here was a portent of a professional triathlon career that had never even occurred to Jacqueline.

When she got to Hawaii, she was not adequately trained for all three events. She had no running background to speak of and only one year on the bicycle. She had never swum competitively before. She wasn't prepared logistically either. She didn't even have swim goggles, and instead of wearing one of the one-piece swimming outfits worn by many female triathletes, she had to wear a bikini. Still, she did well. Emerging from the water in 1:06, she took over the lead at the Hawi turnaround of the bike course and eventually increased her lead to about twenty minutes. She continued to lead until Sylviane and Patricia Puntous passed her at mile 10 of the run. She faded considerably after that, finishing as twenty-first woman.

After the Ironman, Shaw had planned to travel in the South Pacific, but Holiday Health Spa, a workout club, offered to sponsor her, so she did a few more triathlons. Then she was selected for the Canadian National Cycling Team. She rode with the Canadian team in the 1984 Tour de France, the first year the event included a women's division.

Jacqueline believes that the Tour "was one of the best things" she has ever done. She explains: "They treat you incredibly well there, and it's such a big event. People over here don't realize how big the Tour de France is. At the finish line at the Champs Élysées, there must have been two hundred thousand people watching us, a million watching the men."

Jacqueline has become a professional triathlete. In just the first half of the 1985 triathlon season, she competed in sixteen sprint or ultradistance races. She finished first in more than half of those sixteen races, and she has been in the top three in most of them. Shaw has to race a lot because her sole source of income is prize money. Jacqueline reports, "My mom always says, 'When are you going to get a job?' I think I've got a pretty good job." This woman loves what she is doing and does it well.

Jacqueline's close friend and sometime roommate Colleen Cannon also loves being a professional triathlete. Speaking for both, Colleen says, "We like going to work every day." For those two "going to work" means training, traveling, competing, or dealing with publicity chores, although Colleen's work is greatly facilitated by better fortune at finding sponsors. Colleen receives equipment and cash stipends from Nike and Specialized, the bicycle manufacturer. Even in her first major triathlon, the 1983 Ironman, Colleen had financial assistance from Stu and Wendy Hanford, a couple she had met while cycling.

It was at the 1983 Ironman, the first Ironman for both of them, that Colleen and Jacqueline first met. That encounter was brief, but both of them recall that they hit it off immediately. Their shared attitudes about sports, travel, and adventure drew them together. When a mutual friend, veteran triathlete Mark Montgomery, suggested that the three of them live and train together in California, Colleen and Jacqueline readily agreed. As roommates and training partners, Colleen and Jacqueline became firm friends.

Colleen, twenty-four years old, grew up in the flat farm country near Terre Haute, Indiana. She interprets her parents' tennis playing as an influence on her own athletic activity. She has two brothers and two sisters, and between the five Cannon children there always were enough people for a volleyball or basketball game. Her older siblings were active in sports at school, and Colleen followed their example. She started competing in track during the eighth grade. Her junior

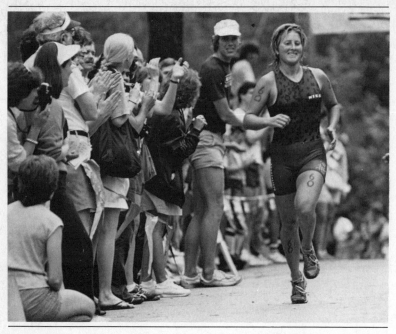

Colleen Cannon at the 1983 Atlanta USTS race.

high school had a girls' athletic association, which introduced the young women of the school to all sorts of sports, even bowling and archery.

Colleen moved from Terre Haute to Auburn, Alabama, during high school. Moving to Alabama initially "was kind of a setback" to her athletic career, she says. It was difficult to participate in athletics in Alabama "because the girls there just don't do too much besides put on a lot of makeup. They're not into working out." She had to overcome peer pressure and lack of opportunity: "I got really ridiculed. They called me a 'jock' and 'the bionic woman.' It was tough being a new person at school, and having to race against the guys because they didn't have a women's track team." She swam competitively during those years only because she was willing to commute to a nearby community for swimming workouts.

When she graduated high school and went on to Auburn University her athletic opportunities improved. As a freshman she made Auburn's varsity swim team, but the long practices interfered with her schoolwork. Colleen had to resign from the swim team, but later during her college career she ran the half mile and 1,500 meters for Auburn's track team. Since she majored in health and physical education she was involved in strenuous activity much of the day, and she also had her track workouts. College summers she worked as a river-raft guide, which fit in nicely with her passion for hiking and back-packing.

Colleen had her first taste of the triathlon during her senior year in college. She competed in the 1983 Oxford Triathlon in Maryland, a relatively long event (2.4-mile swim, 50-mile bike race, 20-mile run). Perhaps Colleen didn't know how to train for a triathlon yet, or possibly she was undertrained. The event was painful for her. Colleen remembers, "I hurt so bad after that race, I couldn't figure out why anybody would do a triathlon. But then the pain went away." The fact that she finished second and attracted the attention of the Specialized bicycle company may have helped chase away the pain. Specialized offered to sponsor her. The company gave her a bicycle to replace the old clunker with baskets she had been riding, and Colleen thought it was the best thing that had ever happened to her.

Apparently, free bicycles are a great tonic, because later that season Cannon entered two more triathlons, USTS events in Tampa and Atlanta. In both of those short-course races she led until near the end, when Sylviane and Patricia Puntous forced her to accept third place. Colleen next tackled the half-Ironman-length Gulf Coast Triathlon, but again she was forced to play third fiddle to the dominant Canadian women.

After she graduated college that summer, Colleen moved to Colorado to train. She lacked the funds to compete, but then Nike came into her life and offered to pay her costs for one race. With the help of the shoe company and her high-altitude training, she took the women's division of the New York USTS race. For her efforts in the Big Apple she picked up a $1,000 prize. Next came Boston's USTS race and another first-place finish. As she readied herself for the 1983 Ironman, she thought she was on a roll.

Unfortunately, things in Kona didn't develop the way she had expected. The Ironman has a way of humbling people. She explains that she was very nervous at the Ironman, missed her food bag on the course, and "bonked" on the bicycle. She was so disappointed with her fourteenth-place finish that she put her bicycle away for many months. After that, she stayed in Hawaii until 1984, working part-time on a charter sailboat.

Her athletic performance and attitude improved substantially in April 1984, when she moved to California to live with Jacqueline Shaw and Mark Montgomery. There, she supported herself with stipends from Nike and Specialized, raced a lot, and won a lot. During 1984 she picked up a great deal of prize money.

Possibly Colleen competed too much in 1984, or possibly she overtrained. During that successful year she often trained fast, with some of the top males in the sport. For many weeks her training regimen included 400 miles of bicycling and 50 miles of running. She swam every single day. Her only breaks from the training routine were races, which were more likely to injure her than allow recuperation of stressed muscles. She says her energy was "just drained." Predictably, she was injured; she pulled a hamstring muscle badly, which set her back for the 1985 season. As this book is being written, she is on the mend and planning for a comeback.

Colleen, Jacqueline, and Dale have some characteristics in common by virtue of sharing both temperament and profession. But female endurance athletes seem to experience the world differently from male endurance athletes. The most glaring dissimilarities between the two female triathletes and Dale are attributable to gender. Jacqueline complains, "I've been told that guys are a wee bit intimidated by us. They don't want to get beat." Dale doesn't necessarily intimidate anyone by being a champion; he just wins the prizes. Jacqueline recalls with a smile, "My mom always told me never to beat a guy arm wrestling; it destroys his ego. I said, 'Well, how about my ego, mom?' " Can you imagine Dale's father telling him not to win at arm wrestling?

Colleen delights in telling the story of the time her friend Jacqueline arm-wrestled a man at a restaurant. The two of them were out for dinner with five other women, and while they were waiting to be seated a muscular fellow was trying to charm Jacqueline into giving him her phone number. The conversation turned to questions of sports and strength. Jacqueline told the guy that she would give him her phone number if he could beat her at arm wrestling. He figured he would win easily, so Jacqueline was able to set the hook. She pointed out that a bet isn't fair unless he put up some stakes too. With scarcely any fear that he would lose, the guy agreed to buy dinner for all seven women if he lost. Colleen reveals the outcome: "She beat that guy! A huge hulk!" Jacqueline says, "I didn't want to pay for dinner, and I didn't want to go out with him anyway."

Another dissimilarity between these female triathletes and Dale is the need to consider security from attack while training. Colleen's father worries about the dangers of her being out on the bike. Jacqueline approaches the security problem by refusing to allow it to circumscribe her activity. She says, "Somebody told me never to ride my bike alone in Southern California. I rode all the way up to Canada. They told me never to go to Venice, in Los Angeles. Man, that's my favorite place!" She thinks that "people are a lot too nervous, and if they show their nervousness it causes problems."

Despite the gender differences, independence is one prominent characteristic that these three professional athletes have in common.

Jacqueline seems to speak for all three when she says, "We couldn't work for too many people now that we've been out on our own for so long." A spirit of adventure is another common thread for the three. Again Jacqueline seems to speak for her colleagues: "There are so many things in the world I would like to try. In my parents' day, if you had more than one job you were considered kind of spacy, because you couldn't hold down a job. Well, society's concept might be changing a bit. There are just too many things out there to stick with one the whole time."

SOME WHO HAVE GREATER BARRIERS

THEY are endurance athletes, too. Some are blind or deaf; some are diabetic; some are epileptic; some have cerebral palsy; some are amputees and wear artificial limbs; some compete in wheelchairs.

These athletes are too varied and unique to be placed in a single category, but they constantly are lumped together under a variety of labels—handicapped, disabled, physically challenged. No one is exactly sure what these terms mean or which are appropriate, especially when applied to athletes. How disabled is a runner with an artificial leg who finishes a marathon ahead of most able-bodied runners? Jim Elliott's epilepsy didn't prevent him from setting a world record by bicycling 502.3 miles in twenty-four hours. On that particular day, Elliott's greatest handicap may have been the strong head winds; he was seeking the record for individual cyclists and therefore couldn't draft in the slipstream of another cyclist.

The concepts of "handicap" and "disability" tend to draw our attention away from the important qualities and achievements of these athletes. Human ingenuity with regard to athletics seems boundless; disabled athletes have invented new sports (such as wheelchair racing) and have made adaptations to existing sports. As we shall see, most of them do not think of themselves as disabled—if anything, they think of themselves just as athletes. Although their disabilities play a role in determining the methods they will use to practice endurance sports, disabled people choose to participate for the same reasons as other athletes: for cardiovascular fitness, to build strength, for recreation, for stress management, to improve self-esteem. And yet it cannot be denied that what these men and women have accomplished is remarkable and worthy of attention because they are, in some way, different.

Some of the best-known disabled athletes are amputees or have lost the normal use of their legs. Perhaps the most famous was Terry Fox, a proud, stubborn, obsessed young Canadian who at the age of eighteen discovered a pain in his right knee that wouldn't go away.

Tests revealed not torn cartilage but a malignant tumor, and doctors amputated Terry's leg just above the knee. He spent painful months in chemotherapy, then learned to play wheelchair basketball. But it wasn't enough.

Terry Fox decided to run. He started by doing laps at a junior high school track in his hometown of Port Coquitlam, a suburb of Vancouver, British Columbia. He built up distance slowly, and had a lighter artificial leg made that he could run on more easily. He entered and finished a marathon; then, as a challenge to himself and to raise money for cancer research, he decided to run 5,000 miles across Canada in the spring of 1980, at a rate of 26 miles a day. He termed his trek a "marathon of hope."

On April 12, Terry dipped his artificial right leg into the Atlantic Ocean at St. John's, Newfoundland, and accompanied by a friend in a van, set off westward. Initially, the weather worked against him. Running long distances was awkward and painful; sometimes his right stump bled.

By the time Terry reached western Quebec, news of his run had begun to spread. When he reached Toronto, Ontario, in June, nearly twenty thousand people turned out to see him. He had become a national hero. Early on, Terry had run alone most of the time. Now it seemed that everyone knew who he was, and he had very little time to call his own.

Terry Fox didn't make it all the way to the Pacific Ocean. His cancer reappeared in his lungs, and he was forced to stop in Thunder Blay, Ontario—3,339 miles from his starting point. He talked of continuing his run when he recovered, but he died less than a year later, in June 1981. He continued to fight until the end, and at the time of his death he had raised $22 million for cancer research. Still more money poured in after his death. "If I die of cancer," Terry Fox said, "I don't want people to forget and say, 'It was a great thing, but now it's over.' I just wish people would remember that anything's possible if you try."

People's lives become entwined in strange and unpredictable ways. Terry Fox, who served as a symbol of hope for so many people, was himself inspired by Dick Traum, who at the New York City Marathon in 1976 became the first runner to complete a marathon with an artificial leg. Fox had kept a picture of Dick Traum by his bed before the operation in which his leg was amputated, and after the operation he met with Traum, who encouraged him to do his trans-Canada run.

Dick Traum, now forty-four, was struck from behind by an automobile in 1964 while he was putting gas in his own car at a service station. His right leg was crushed and had to be amputated. After spending a year in a wheelchair, Traum was fitted with an artificial leg. He was overweight and, in an attempt to do something about that, enrolled in an ordinary fitness class at New York City's West Side YMCA. Bob Glover headed that class. Because the other—nondisabled—people in the class ran, Traum ran too. He saw nothing unusual about that, although he later discovered that at the time he was probably the only person in the country running on an artificial leg.

Eventually, Traum decided to run a marathon. He began the 1976 New York City race four hours ahead of two thousand other runners. The picture of him running that marathon—the first of six in New York City—appeared in newspapers and running magazines, and made the general public aware that endurance sports could be undertaken and mastered by disabled athletes.

In 1983, Traum got together with Glover, who by then had written several books on running, and the New York Road Runners Club, to found the Achilles Track Club for disabled runners. The idea was that anyone could participate, regardless of previous athletic background, as long as he or she was disabled. The club started slowly, but now has a membership of more than eighty athletes who have all kinds of disabilities: blindness, cerebral palsy, paralysis, strokes, cancer, amputation, polio. Membership in the club is free.

Achilles Club workouts are held each Wednesday at 6:30 P.M. at the International Running Center on East Eighty-ninth Street in Manhattan, headquarters of the New York Road Runners Club. Traum coaches, as do national-class masters runner Patty Lee Parmalee, several physical therapists, and a wheelchair trainer. Workouts consist of warmup and stretching; outdoor training around the Central Park reservoir; nutrition, health, and equipment information; and individual training advice.

The philosophy of the Achilles Track Club is that anyone can do something and, given the opportunity and proper guidance, most people can do more than they think they can. Although each member works out his or her individual goals, thirteen club members started and finished the 1984 New York City Marathon.

One of those club members was Linda Down, twenty-eight, who has cerebral palsy. She and her twin sister, Laura, who also has cerebral palsy, had watched the 1981 marathon on television in their Manhattan apartment. In the spring of 1982, Linda finished work on a research grant and found herself unemployed. Like many incipient athletes, she wanted to lose some weight and improve her general physical condition. She started doing sit-ups, and then thought she'd try to run.

Running, for Linda Down, means planting the rubber tips of her crutches on the ground in front of her, leaning forward, lifting her body weight, and swinging/dragging first her left and then her right leg under and then ahead of her upper body. She uses what are termed Canadian forearm crutches, which have supports under the elbows rather than under the upper arms.

Linda entered the L'Eggs Mini-Marathon, May 1982, finishing the 10-kilometer course in two hours. She increased her training, doing up to seven-hour workouts—16 to 18 miles—on Fifth Avenue sidewalks, aiming for the October marathon. In the 1982 New York City Marathon, Down started with the other runners and finished in the darkness, eleven hours and fifteen minutes later. In the last half of the race, she was accompanied by her mother and sister in a car, and by the ABC camera crew, who told the story of her struggle to American television viewers. As a result, Linda Down was invited to the White House to meet with President Reagan, along with race winners Alberto Salazar and Grete Waitz.

Since that race, Down has found employment as the first director of Disabled Students' Services at Adelphi University, where she had earned a master's degree in social work. She also has stuck with and improved her running. She was inspired by the creation of the Achilles Track Club and became one of its first five members. In 1983, she started with Traum three hours in front of the other runners and lowered her time to 8:45. In 1984, she set a personal record despite breaking a crutch toward the end of the marathon. Down has lowered her 10-kilometer pace to 14:30 per mile, has lost thirty pounds, and has developed some power in her legs.

Patrick Griskus, thirty-seven, of Waterbury, Connecticut, also a member of the Achilles Track Club, is the world's fastest amputee runner. Griskus lost his left leg just below the knee in the Marine Corps in 1967, when he hit a car head-on while riding his motorcycle. Always a good athlete—he'd run a 4:28 mile and a 9.8 100-yard dash in school—Griskus had some bad times, including problems with abuse of alcohol, before returning to running in 1981. Since then, the muscular five-foot-eleven, 150-pound athlete has come back with a vengeance. He began running marathons in 1983 and set a personal record at Boston in 1984 with a 3:44.30.

In 1984, Pat Griskus began doing triathlons. On September 8, he lined up with 270 other athletes at the start of the Cape Cod Endurance Triathlon, which consisted of Ironman distances in the swim, bike, and run. He finished the 2.4-mile swim in 1:45—in 61-degree water—took just over 6:30 to cycle 112 miles, then tightened up in the marathon, finishing the event in 14:28.57, a time many able-bodied athletes would be pleased to claim. Griskus swims regularly, cycles 200 miles a week, and runs 60 miles a week. "Because I'm an amputee, many people think that it's enough that I just show up and finish races," Griskus says. "I can't see that there's anything right in that attitude. I compete against time and as many people as I can beat."

Bill Carlson, who has diabetes, shares the same focus as Griskus. He also expresses more concern for his triathlon performance than he does for his handicap. After an outstanding ninth place finish out of a field of three hundred at the 1984 Mighty Hamptons Triathlon, he told filmmaker Ambrose Salmini, "It seems that I have such good control of my diabetes. There's nothing that's going to stop me now. I'm just going to continue to train and become a better athlete." In the 1985 Ironman, Carlson achieved his goal of finishing before dark.

Lance Younger, twenty-eight, lives in Seal Beach in Southern California. He lost his left leg below the knee in a motorcycle accident when he was nineteen. Younger excels in triathlons of all distances, often placing in the top 10 percent of the field, but his specialty seems to be the ultras. He placed thirty-fourth out of several hundred triathletes in the Ironman-length Los Angeles Centurion Triathlon in 1983.

Younger uses a special prosthesis that consists of a steel shaft attached to the pedal of his bicycle on a ball-and-socket joint. On the top of the shaft is a fiberglass cup that holds his leg in place. Unlike Pat Griskus, Lance runs in a wheelchair instead of using an artificial leg.

Lance considers 1983 a "learning year," in which his goal was to gain experience in triathlons. The high point of his 1984 season had to be his first-place finish at the King of the Hill Long Course (97 miles) at California's Big Bear Lake, which he won over Gary Hooker by a margin of forty-eight seconds. He passed Hooker with less than 200 yards to go—after more than seven and a half hours of racing—but refused to accept the win, stating that his wheelchair gave him an unfair advantage. Race organizers named Younger and Hooker co-winners of the event.

Of all disabled athletes, perhaps the most controversial are wheelchair racers, at least as far as "mainstreaming" is concerned—that is, participating in races with able-bodied runners. Some race organizers and runners consider the presence of wheelchair racers hazardous to the well-being of able-bodied runners; the chairs sometimes reach speeds of close to 50 miles per hour.

Wheelchair racers were not officially recognized at Boston until 1984, and the New York City Marathon went to court to exclude wheelchair racers. Although the New York Marathon won its point after a lengthy court battle, New York Mayor Edward Koch threatened to bar the use of the public streets unless the event included wheelchair athletes. The compromise that eventually emerged permits wheelchair

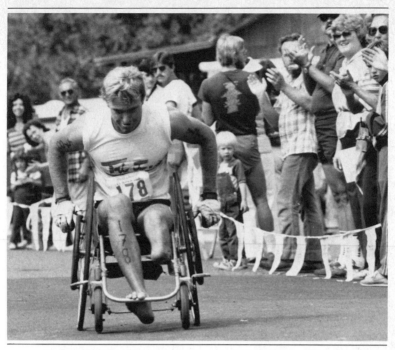

Lance Younger completing a USTS triathlon.
COURTESY OF BUD LIGHT USTS

racers to participate, but does not give them a separate division or starting time. Without independent status, relatively few wheelchair athletes enter the New York marathon. In general, though, wheelchair racers are now accepted in more events.

This is good news for Jim Knaub, twenty-nine, of Long Beach, California. Knaub is a handsome, articulate, outspoken world-class athlete who has run the marathon in 1:47.10—twenty minutes faster than the fastest runner—in his racing wheelchair.

Jim Knaub has been an athlete most of his life. He was a national-class pole vaulter for Long Beach State University in the mid-seventies and a semifinalist at the 1976 Olympic trials. A traffic accident with a drunk driver in 1978 left him paralyzed from the waist down. While completing a rehabilitation program in a Los Angeles hospital, Knaub saw wheelchair racer Bob Hall run the 1978 New York City Marathon and decided to start racing.

Primarily a marathoner, Knaub trains 20 to 30 miles a day when he can put in the time. Typically, he might work out in the morning with a 17- to 20-mile run along the flood-control canals or on Pacific Coast Highway south from his Long Beach apartment. In the evening he tries to get in 10 miles on the track or on an ergometer; Knaub also works out on Nautilus equipment.

Knaub set two national marks while competing in the California Wheelchair Games in April 1984. He lowered the 5,000-meter record by twenty-four seconds with a 14:53.8, and also took almost a second off the record for 800 meters, running a 2:17.44. Knaub has won the Boston Marathon twice, in 1982 and 1983 (when he ran his 1:47.10). In 1985, he was third (1:48.44) in a disputed race at Boston, behind American George Murray (1:45.34) and Canadian Andre Viger (1:47.33).

Besides being an athlete, Jim Knaub has worked as a television actor, but most of his other professional time is spent working as a performance and products consultant and program specialist for Invacare Corporation, a manufacturer of wheelchairs and other medical equipment based in Elyria, Ohio. "Most chairs have been designed by able-bodied people," he says. "It's my job to go out and gather information about what features ought to be put into a chair and to work with the design engineers on that, so that guys in chairs don't have to get out hacksaws and cut up and reweld chairs so that they work." Knaub works on chair design for both wheelchair athletes and others restricted to wheelchairs.

In 1984, Knaub "trained down" (changed his stroke, did more anaerobic work) to the 1,500 meters so that he could compete on August 11 in an exhibition event at the Los Angeles Olympic Games. Eight men raced their wheelchairs at 1,500 meters and eight women raced theirs at 800 meters. Knaub was undefeated all year in the 1,500, but "crashed in his second race" at the trials held a few weeks before in New York, and failed to make the finals in Los Angeles. "The '84 Games were the first time in the history of the Olympics that they've had anything for wheelchairs. We don't know what's going to happen in 1988 at Seoul, but we're working so that there will be other events for people in chairs."

One of the most versatile endurance athletes with a disability is Harry Cordellos, forty-seven, a lifelong resident of San Francisco. Cordellos was born blind and, as a child, had eight operations on his eyes that gave him partial vision. During high school his sight began to worsen, and he had six more operations to try to save it. The world became like a fog to Harry Cordellos—"a fog that never lifted," as he describes it in his autobiography, *Breaking Through*. He accepted the fact that he eventually would become totally blind and began to learn how to be self-sufficient at the Oakland Orientation Center for the Blind after graduating from high school.

One particular event changed Harry's life completely. He had never been particularly athletic, and during his last year or so of high school, he had become quite depressed and withdrawn. A shop instructor at the Center for the Blind, Everett Whitney, took Harry and several other blind students for a weekend of camping and recreation at a lake near San Francisco. Though totally blind, Harry astonished himself by learning to water-ski. "If I can water-ski," he said to himself, "I can do anything." Today, nearly thirty years later, water-skiing remains his favorite sport.

As he pursued a college degree, Harry found his interest in athletics growing. He learned to dive and swim, and he began running regularly as a senior at Cal State College in Hayward. He found that he enjoyed running in races such as the San Francisco Bay-to-Breakers, which he has run every year since 1968. Before long, Harry succumbed to another "illness"—marathon fever. He ran his first, San Francisco's Golden Gate Marathon, in 1970, and he has run more than sixty since, including several at Boston. His marathon best is 2:57.42, and he runs six to eight each year.

Harry's athletic achievements don't stop there. He completed Hawaii's Ironman Triathlon in 1981 in a time of 16:26.17 on minimal training—he swam and bicycled only four times each in the several months preceding the race. In 1980, he became the first blind skier to participate in the American Birkebeiner 55-kilometer cross-country ski race in Telemark, Wisconsin. He has also run the infamous Dipsea and Double Dipsea races on Mount Tamalpais in Marin County, north of San Francisco, several times. An award-winning film, *Survival Run,* was made about one of those Dipsea attempts.

Harry has also cycled the Davis (California) Double Century and the Spenco 500 in Waco, Texas, and he has water-skiied from Santa Catalina Island to the Queen Mary in Long Beach, California, 31 miles away.

Because he is blind, Harry must train and race with sighted partners. He runs by keeping light contact with his partner's hand or forearm, listening to verbal cues to negotiate curves or avoid obstacles. On rugged cross-country runs such as the Dipsea, he wears gloves and knee pads and, on rough and downhill sections, holds on to his partner's hips or elbows from behind, in what he calls a "choo-choo-train" style. While swimming he is guided by a partner on a surfboard, and he cycles on the back of a tandem. (Blind athletes have used some other clever adaptations to enable them to enjoy endurance sport. For example, in 1946 a blind swimmer from Hawaii, King Benny Nawahi, swam the 23-mile Catalina Channel using a system somewhat like a submarine's sonar. He followed the sound of the bell on board his pilot boat).

For several years, Harry worked for BART (Bay Area Rapid Transit), giving customers route and travel information. Now, he works as a motivational lecturer and workshop consultant in physical education. (He has a master's degree in physical education.) His future athletic goals include running the original marathon course in Greece (his family is Greek), running several more sub-three-hour marathons, and improving his time on the Santa Catalina–to–Queen Mary water-ski trip.* "Sports has changed my attitude toward myself," Harry has said. "I'm more accepted in sports than anywhere else. Besides, I think I've proved that blindness isn't that limited a condition."

The United States Association of Blind Athletes, headquartered in Beach Haven Park, New Jersey, would heartily agree with Harry. It is the goal of that nonprofit, volunteer organization to promote opportunities for blind athletes to train and compete in a wide variety of athletic activities, including such endurance sports as running, skiing, and swimming. And many blind athletes do just that.

THE INSPIRATION FALLACY

Jim Knaub, world-class wheelchair racer, says, "The biggest problem we have to overcome is the public's ignorance." The truth is, as Knaub points out, most people never really look at disabled athletes, or if they do, they see what they want to see. This is understandable; if you're able-bodied, it's difficult to look at and think about someone who is blind or missing a leg, because the natural initial reaction is fear: "God, I don't know what I'd do if that happened to me!"

Experiencing injuries can make athletes particularly afraid of the fate of the disabled. In June 1985 Pat Griskus told *Ultrasport* magazine that, "Everybody has injuries that hinder their performance at one time or another. In that sense we're all in the same boat." Of course, most sidelined athletes recover or can easily change to another sport that doesn't use the injured body parts. Such athletic injuries usually don't interfere with day-to-day life, and they only rarely are stigmatizing, because they are not visible to others. Candace Cable, a wheelchair racer and competitive swimmer, whose paralysis was caused by the criminal negligence of a drunken motorist, goes straight to the heart of the fear: "We're all only able-bodied temporarily. Sooner or later everyone's body breaks down." That is an unpleasant realization that the able-bodied would rather avoid.

Hence, most people react to disabled athletes as they might react to someone they've been told has terminal cancer: with an uneasy mixture of concern, respect, sympathy, sorrow, and awe. The sense of awe is heightened and the sorrow diminished, of course, be-

---

*In the summer of 1985, while this book was in preparation, Cordellos again skied the Catalina Channel and accomplished his mission. He crossed the Channel in one hour and twenty-eight minutes, decreasing his previous best by more than half.

cause the disabled athlete is usually in excellent health and not about to die.

So it becomes easy to see the disabled athlete as "inspirational," which in and of itself is not a distorted or demeaning perception. To see Harry Cordellos run the Dipsea race, which is difficult enough for a sighted person, *is* inspirational, and it's entirely appropriate to react by thinking, Wow! If someone who can't see can do that race, I can probably do a whole lot more than I'm doing. Indeed, both individual disabled athletes and organizations representing disabled athletes have been inspired by the examples of others who are disabled: Terry Fox was inspired by Dick Traum, and the motto of the National Handicapped Sports and Recreation Association (shown across a picture of a one-legged water-skier) is "If I Can Do This, I Can Do Anything!" Griskus believes that it is good to genuinely inspire others, but for him consciously projecting himself as a model involves "far too much self-serving hoopla."

The difficulty in dealing candidly with disabled people in general and with disabled athletes in particular is reflected in the terminology we use to discuss the issue. The two terms in most current usage to describe the athletes found in this chapter are "handicapped" and "disabled." "Handicapped" is the older term, and the one under which someone doing library research will find the most information—it's the term used in Library of Congress subject headings, for example. And yet it's also the term in greatest disfavor, excluding such obviously inaccurate labels as "crippled," "deformed," and "abnormal." For most people, "disabled" seems to be the most neutral and acceptable adjective, the one with the least negative connotation. "Physically challenged," the term that became popular at the Los Angeles Olympics, strikes many people as a stilted euphemism.

There is no general agreement among athletes about what terms are best, either. Knaub, for example, feels strongly that "handicapped" is a negative term, calling to mind someone with cap in hand looking for a handout. But Harry Cordellos says, "Any way you look at it, I'm handicapped. A handicap is a condition that makes a job more difficult, and there's no question that being blind makes my life more difficult. And in one sense, it's inaccurate to say I'm a disabled runner, because that makes me sound like I can't run. But I *am* a runner with a disability."

The difficulty of finding language to deal with the realities of the disabled points to two important truths: language is imprecise and the subject of disabled athletes is an emotional one. Suppose you're an able-bodied runner in a 10-kilometer race and you see someone running the race beside you who's in a wheelchair or who has an artificial leg. How do you somehow acknowledge that that runner is different from most people and that the event may be more difficult for him or her—without being condescending or distorting what's important and true about that runner's life? What words do you use?

There are no easy answers. At one extreme disabled athletes—blind runners, wheelchair racers, amputee triathletes—have been lumped together within a category that has ignored their individual differences. The focus has been on the disability, not on the situation of the individual athlete who happens to be disabled. At the other extreme, disabled athletes have been "invisible." "Take the Perrier 10-K," says Jim Knaub. "I've paid my $15 there for years; they've given me a number, but they've never had a wheelchair division."

Both approaches have resulted in distortion, in what Knaub called "the public's ignorance." Linda Down told *Runner's World,* "I don't think disabled people are represented as people with the same feelings and aspirations as everyone else. You only see disabled people on telethons . . . but never in the day-to-day kinds of things that everyone else does. The image you have is not of the person, but of the disability."

Disabled athletes *don't* see themselves as particularly inspirational or courageous, for example, although that seems to be one of the dominant impressions the general public has of them. "I feel uncomfortable when people tell me I'm courageous," Down says of public reaction to her dealing with cerebral palsy. "To me, there's no other choice. If I had the choice of sitting in my apartment and looking at four walls or going out and doing something that I wanted to do, I'd simply go out and do it. Anybody faced with the same circumstances would probably do the same thing."

In fact *all* endurance athletes, including disabled ones, have done exactly what Down has; they've risked failure by going out and doing something. Taking that risk first involves overcoming the handicap that *all* humans share to some degree—low self-confidence. Since disabled athletes must also conquer society's doubts about their ability, non-handicapped people—who may be suffering from some lack of self-confidence—are naturally impressed by the handicapped athlete, who has that much more to overcome. So the tag of "inspirational" is hard for the disabled athlete to shake.

Being considered inspirational has somewhat different consequences for elite athletes like Knaub. "We're treated differently than other athletes," he says. "Nobody points at a Salazar and says, 'Isn't he inspirational?' They say, 'Isn't he incredible?' We want that said about us. People don't realize how much work goes into what we do."

COMPETING IN THE MAINSTREAM

Elite able-bodied athletes often can make a living from their sport, but that is not so for the disabled athlete. "In the militant years, we used to try to prove ourselves *against* the runners," says Knaub. "Now, we realize we're racing along *with* them. Still, a Rodgers or a Dixon gets ten or fifteen grand to show up at a race, pick his nose, and jog across the finish line. We're sick and tired of people *just* saying, 'Isn't he inspirational?' We're saying, 'Yeah, but we want the paycheck, too!' "

Knaub knows that it's not entirely a matter of distorted perceptions. "I realize that running is a business," he says, "and that chair racers haven't got the numbers. We can't get sixty thousand chairs to a race. The biggest have seventy chairs, so we can't ask for $20,000. But we can ask for *something*. All we're asking for is a little respect for what we get out there and do."

Disabled athletes *are* getting more respect and encouragement than they have in the past. It wasn't so long ago—about forty years— that any sport for the disabled was considered strictly therapy, not competition. Then disabled American soldiers of World War II informally began playing wheelchair basketball at Veteran's Administration hospitals. The first organized wheelchair sports event in Europe was the Stoke-Mandeville Games, held in England in 1948. There were only twenty-six participants, all from England, and a few events (shotput, javelin, club throw, and archery) in those first games. Since 1952, the annual Stoke-Mandeville Games have become an international competition.

Today, dozens of organizations exist to encourage and support disabled athletes at all levels, in a variety of sports ranging from cross-country skiing to swimming to track and field. A major symbolic breakthrough occurred in 1984, when world champion wheelchair marathoner George Murray became the first disabled athlete to appear on the front of the Wheaties box. Consumers had selected Murray and five other nondisabled athletes in a national poll.

Some countries have taken progressive positions with respect to the support of disabled athletes. Perhaps the most noteworthy is Canada. Its Athlete Assistance Program defrays much of the training and competition expenses, without discriminating between able-bodied and disabled athletes. Recognizing that certain expenses increase as higher standards of international performance are achieved, Canadian athletes are given A, B, or C "cards" (a method of classification) based on performance and potential in their sport. The focus is on Olympic sports, but there is a wheelchair division in the international classification. The top athletes, able-bodied and disabled, receive a living and training stipend. In the wheelchair category (A and B carding), there are ten cards available (eight men, two women); four are for the marathon. "Our goal is to provide the same level of support as able-bodied athletes get," says Andy Fleming of the Canadian National Wheelchair Athletic Association. "We want equal service, not special service."

Disabled athletes occasionally are so competent in their sport that in some situations they forget they're not part of the mainstream. For instance, Jim Penseyres, who is now a machinist by trade, lost his left leg below the knee when as a Marine in Vietnam he stepped on a land mine. In 1984, Jim was a member of the support crew for his older brother, Pete, in the 3,047-mile Race Across AMerica (RAAM). Since Jim is a competitive cyclist (he cycles with a prosthesis) it is quite understandable that the bug would bite him to be a contestant in the 1985 RAAM. His training included a fifth-place finish at the 325-mile Arizona Challenge, which includes 18,000 feet of vertical climb. The day after that event Jim and some companions were on their way to a restaurant. Unfortunately, the famished group was having difficulty finding a parking place at the shopping mall where the restaurant was located. As they cruised the lot, one of his companions pointed to a space marked "handicapped" and said, "Let's park there." Without thinking Jim automatically responded, "We can't, that's for handicapped." Although he had lost his leg many years earlier, it had not occurred to Jim that his disability might make him eligible to use a handicapped parking place.

In general, disabled athletes are gaining greater recognition and acceptance in organized athletic events. The New York City Marathon is about the only major running event that has tried to prevent mass participation by wheelchairs. More typical is the creation of a wheelchair triathlon by the Dallas Park and Recreation Department, which consists of rafting, pushing (running), and swimming events. There is a short and a long course, and a "superstar" competition as well. The Dallas triathlon has been conducted for three years. And in 1985, Invacare, the wheelchair and medical equipment firm for which Jim Knaub works, sponsored a seven-race "Invacare Cup Series" of road-racing events, to be held at seven of the top races in the United States, including the Lilac Bloomsday Run, the Kaiser Roll, the *Detroit Free Press* Marathon, the Long Beach Half-Marathon, and the Orange Bowl Marathon. Total prize money for the series is $150,000.

Acceptance of the disabled athlete by other athletes and spectators (as opposed to event promoters) has often been high. As Harry Cordellos says, "I've been more accepted in sports than anywhere else."

Indeed, as more and more disabled persons become athletes, the most important truth will become evident: what sets the disabled athletes apart is that they are athletes, not that they are disabled. In some ways, the disability normalizes the disabled athletes, forcing them to deal with the limitations imposed by their disabilities and to transcend them.

"My biggest disability is that I'm an athlete," says Jim Knaub. "I've had to make a lot of sacrifices to become one. Financially, I'd be doing better, I'd be able to devote more time to a career. Being an athlete limits the amount of time you can devote to relationships. Being an athlete affects my life more than being in a chair."

But Knaub, like able-bodied athletes, accepts the consequences of his choice. "A man is what he thinks about all day," he says. "Most of the true athletes I know, wheelchair or not, constantly think about their sport."

THE MOTIVATION

PART

3

POSITIVE MOTIVATIONS: THE BRIGHT SIDE OF SPORTS

A RATHER DOUR graduate student in California wears a T-shirt that carries the slogan "Life is hard, then you die." To many people the grim words on that shirt sum up the world view of endurance athletes. Most people in our society have other occupations and preoccupations that compete for the time required by endurance training. Why does the endurance athlete do it?

Some athletes blithely say, "Because it's there." That statement—often misattributed to Sir Edmund Hillary—was George L. Mallory's way of evading the question of why he wanted to climb Mount Everest. Mallory, who died during his attempt on Everest, was no doubt trying to say that he couldn't understand, much less explain, his own motivation.

When pressed to probe deeper, most endurance athletes admit that their motivations are complex, and they have come up with a variety of reasons. Mixed in with the many contradictory answers are a few that seem eminently reasonable.

PLAIN OLD FUN

Almost universally, endurance athletes object vigorously to any suggestion that they are masochistic. True, you often will hear long-distance swimmers, cyclists, runners, or rowers grouse about a particularly painful race, then later describe their experiences in nostalgic, positive terms. Yet they don't train or compete to bask in their misery. On the contrary, many say they train hard in order to be more comfortable when competing. Endurance athletes do not necessarily love pain; rather, they are willing to withstand some misery in pursuit of their goals.

Curiously, though training injuries and overtraining are common, athletes usually don't refer to training as painful. Possibly the absence of the immediate incentives offered by competition keeps athletes from going beyond the pain threshold during training. It is not torture.

177

Pushing all out in an event often is perceived as painful, but training almost never. In fact, amateur endurance athletes either complain about the responsibilities that interfere with training, or express guilt about neglecting their duties and chores because they prefer to train. Professional endurance athletes frequently say that they chose their occupation because it is one of the few ways they know to get paid for having fun.

"A lot of people I know go out and run because they think it's good for them or because they want to lose weight," says Brian, an amateur triathlete. "It's tough for them, because they're not having fun with it. I like doing all this stuff. It's easy to get up the ambition to go for a bicycle ride, or go for a swim, or go for a run, because if you enjoy it, you don't really mind doing it. You look forward to it."

So, far from being an expression of masochism, the motivation to engage in endurance athletics simply may be pleasure seeking. Those who participate in a sport perceive it as entertainment, even though someone else might call it self-punishment.

NEEDS AS MOTIVATION

Harvard University psychology professor David McClelland has dedicated his life to studying motivation. He developed a means to assess human motivation that he calls the Thematic Aperception Test, or TAT. In the TAT a person is asked to write a story about a picture whose meaning is purposely ambiguous. According to McClelland, the response one gives to the ambiguous stimulus is indicative of one's needs. Many psychologists and also folk wisdom suggest that unfulfilled needs motivate behavior; e.g., I am thirsty—an indication that I need water—therefore I drink.

McClelland's research has identified various nonphysiological needs that seem to underlie the TAT stories that people write. The three principal needs in McClelland's motivation theory are the need for affiliation, the need for achievement, and the need for power. By affiliation McClelland means social interaction, love, affection, feelings of belongingness, and friendship. Thus, any references to a social or family relationship in a TAT story may be evidence of a person's need for affiliation. McClelland's need for achievement includes a desire to build things or be creative. A story in which one of the characters may lead or direct one of the other characters suggests that the writer has some need for power. The proportions of relevant themes in a person's stories supposedly determine the extent to which that person is motivated by need for affiliation, achievement, or power. Of course, individuals vary greatly in what motivates them, as they do in their scores on the scales of McClelland's test.

One could debate forever whether McClelland's test validly measures the three types of motivation. Leaving that question aside, however, common sense suggests that unfulfilled needs for affiliation, achievement, or power are likely to be strong motivators. The presence of any one of those three needs could explain the drive to participate in endurance athletics.

For instance, if a sport is pursued regularly, it quickly becomes intertwined in a person's social life. Athletes meet other people while practicing their sport and that leads to friendships. Friends who share an interest in a given endurance sport often influence each other to try greater challenges. Alex, an ultradistance runner who trained with his son for the Ironman Triathlon, thinks he was motivated by wanting to be close to his son. Lois trained for the Ironman-length Cape Cod Endurance Triathlon with her brother, Larry, and she says, "I just don't think I could have motivated myself . . . to do those 70-mile bike rides alone." Hence, the sport can become a focal point of activity and social interaction, helping to fulfill the need for affiliation.

A person who can run or ski cross-country for 10 kilometers may well be motivated to increase the level of exertion and run a marathon or ski the 55-kilometer Birkebeiner, adding new achievements to his or her credit. Also, quite frequently endurance athletes have already been successful in their occupations or avocations, and they perceive athletic contests as another opportunity to excel. Endurance athletes often seem to look for greater challenges almost as soon as they have achieved their current goals. That is why the existence of endurance triathlons that dwarf the formidable Ironman does not seem surprising. For many endurance athletes the need for achievement may explain much of their motivation.

The need for power may also make sense here. If you are an endurance athlete, you probably know that competition is often a major motivator. Alternatively, you may believe that you are not interested in measuring yourself against your peers: but rest assured that some of your peers are interested in measuring themselves against you. For many endurance athletes—as for many people of all sorts—the need for power is an important motivator. Power goes beyond just attaining superiority over others in a competition. The need for power can encompass a need for mastery over the event itself. Few activities more directly fulfill a need for a feeling of mastery than overcoming a purely physical challenge.

Modern American life has robbed most of us of the life-and-death challenges that our ancestors routinely faced. Obviously, some of us have occupations that affect the health and safety of our communities. But few of us are truly essential; somebody else would take over if the job is critical to the maintenance of life or social order. Fewer still would find their own survival immediately threatened if they didn't do their job next week, next month, or perhaps all next year. True, sooner or later deserters from the economic battlefield have to find new work or at least apply for welfare, but for the most part our physical survival doesn't depend on continuously working at the same task. The safety net is usually there. That was not true just one or two hundred years ago. In years gone by, farmers who didn't plant their crops might begin starving to death by harvest time. Since daily existence rarely provides the life-and-death challenges it once did, many twentieth-century Americans may feel deprived of meaningful goals. Many people compensate for the loss of survival challenge by engaging in all manner of creative endeavor in art, science, literature, and sport. In short, many individuals have become endurance athletes in order to give themselves the goals their lives would otherwise lack.

Champion marathon swimmer Jon Erikson, now a salesman for Motorola, puts it this way: "Life's nothing without a goal, whether to swim the Channel, write a book, or sell a lot of two-way radios. We have to have goals because if we cease to have them we may as well give it up." Confucius reputedly said that a man without a goal is like a ship without a rudder. What better rudder than an endurance challenge?

FEELINGS OF COMPETENCE AND MASTERY

Athletes often report substantial boosts to their feelings of competence after successfully completing endurance events. In some cases descriptions of those feelings border on arrogance. (Endurance athletes sometimes express feelings of superiority over those who are sedentary.) Many men and women pursue endurance athletics because it makes them feel self-reliant to know that whenever they might need to or want to they could comfortably maintain a high level of exertion for a long period of time. The competent feel secure, self-confident, and self-possessed.

Success in difficult endurance events profoundly affects one's feelings of self-confidence. Mary Ann, a triathlete, expressed it this way: "After I did the first Ironman, something might come up that would be a little bit hard. I'd start to say, 'Ooh, I can't do that.' But then I'd say, 'Of course I can. If I can do the Ironman, of course I can do this.' " For many twentieth-century Americans, marathons and triathlons are rites of passage that test one's mettle.

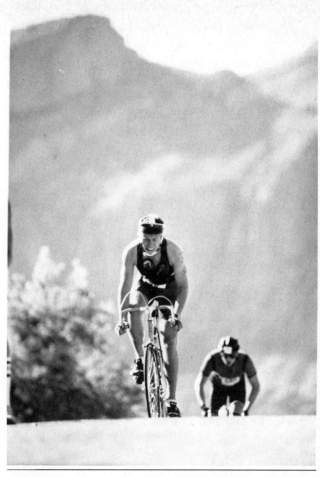

Cresting a monstrous hill at the Fountain Mountain Triathlon certainly represents a challenge.

PHOTO BY BUDD SYMES

In its advertising, the U.S. Marine Corps trades heavily on the need to find tests for one's competence. Well, it's not just the Marine Corps that builds men; the triathlon builds men too. One athlete, who does well in the masters (over forty) division of triathlons, says, "I know the word *validation* is a cliché, but it is a validation of a certain sort to know that I can go out there with my age mates, and I don't have to make any apologies. I'm a competitor. I can stay right in there with the best of them." In a world that places us increasingly at the mercy of giant bureaucracies and dehumanizing machines, it's wonderful to find activities that restore our feelings of raw, individual potency.

More than "just" feelings of competence are involved in this, though. For any of us, perhaps all of us, the situation may well arise in which endurance can make the difference between life and death. On some level—in our nightmares, if nowhere else—we are probably all aware that such dire situations may arise. Your auto breaks down on the desert; as an endurance athlete you know that you can walk, perhaps run, to the next town. That subliminal awareness may be the cause of much anxiety, and proving one's competence in endurance athletics goes a long way toward allaying those feelings.

HEALTH AND FITNESS

In the past decade physical fitness has become a national obsession. We are inundated with fitness propaganda. At an early morning hour, when the psyche is particularly susceptible to recommendations, the face of football coach George Allen beams out from the back of the cornflakes box, urging us, on behalf of the President's Council on Physical Fitness, to get out there with our stopwatches and put our children through rigorous fitness tests. The popularity of fitness books is one tangible consequence of the obsession. Another is the phenomenal growth of athletic shoe companies. Nike grew from zero to $867 million annual sales in only twenty years. And participation in endurance sport has blossomed. Twenty-five years ago the fitness center industry hardly existed. Now you have to reserve long in advance to get a lane at the lap pool or a racquetball court during peak hours.

Almost certainly the pro-fitness propaganda serves a very desirable purpose. There is substantial evidence that physical fitness promotes health, and many people are motivated by this to become endurance athletes. Perhaps they were out of shape and overweight until they began a program of running, swimming, or some other aerobic exercise. Possibly they took up aerobic activity for reasons of vanity; athletes look good. They have slim, well-toned bodies, clear complexions, and a general appearance of health. Once they have experienced the initial benefits of their fitness program, they graduated to endurance sport.

Related to the fitness motivation is that of overcoming a specific health problem. The author of *The Joy of Running*, Thaddeus Kostrubala, exemplifies this sort of motivation. He had been diagnosed as a high-risk candidate for cardiovascular disease when he enrolled in John Boyer's exercise program for recuperating heart patients at San Diego State University. Cris, from southern California, had heart surgery and became an endurance athlete as a result of his efforts to recuperate. One must ease into such programs very gradually, and that is what Cris did. Beginning with short walks, under close medical supervision, he built up to the point where he could comfortably complete marathons, and after ten years he still runs long distances virtually every day. Sue, who lives in central Texas, had surgery at ten years old to correct a congenital heart defect. As an adult she has become an avid bicyclist and runner. Sue plans to participate in a 500-mile bicycle race next fall.

Another athlete, Howard, was institutionalized for many years as a schizophrenic. Upon his release in the early 1970s he became a runner; he believes it was a spontaneous way to work out his nervous tension. Initially obese, Howard trimmed down to a lean 150 pounds and steadily increased his running, at one point getting up to over 100 miles per week. He quit smoking and took himself off medication. He met and befriended numerous other runners in his local community, and at one point of his athletic career Howard was regularly running marathons at speeds as low as two hours and thirty-four minutes. There are many mementos and trophies at his house from the short and long footraces in which he has been the overall or age-group winner. Howard still runs, but he has decreased his weekly mileage to about 40, and now he also bicycles and occasionally works out at a gym. His psychiatric problems have never returned, he is happily married, holds down a steady job, and has many friends.

Fred, an ultradistance rower, speaks for many endurance enthusiasts when he says that he began rowing as a way to cope with stress. He says it is impossible for him to dwell on stressful problems while he is engaged in a strenuous workout. More than fifty years ago medical researcher Dr. Hans Selye suggested that the stress of life interferes with the immune response and is implicated as a cause of numerous ailments. In particular, stress is now thought to have a role in heart disease. According to Fred, the problems that earlier seemed so thorny always appear much less difficult when his workout is finished. As he says, "How important could the problems be if I forget them during the exertion?" His endurance training doesn't solve the problems, but he believes it diminishes their secondary effects.

Still, exercise is not a panacea. Cris, the heart surgery survivor, strictly adheres to the Pritikin diet and carefully limits his intake of cholesterol. Both Howard and Fred have friendships, good marriages, and generally healthy life-styles to help them maintain their mental and physical health. Their exercise is part of a healthful plan, not the entire solution. There is no way to *prove* that endurance athletics by itself will take care of a given health problem, but it certainly appears that a desire to improve or maintain good health has motivated many people to participate in endurance athletics.

Another motivation for the endurance athlete is the desire to prove the doctor wrong. Theodore Roosevelt allegedly climbed the Matterhorn soon after being told by his physician that he had a "weak heart." Of course, this book does not recommend that readers disregard medical advice. The procedures have improved considerably since the nineteenth century, when Roosevelt was probably misdiagnosed. Still, as risky or foolish as it may be, some people have sought endurance challenges as a way to express defiance against the death sentence imposed by the diagnosis of a terminal ailment, just as Teddy Roosevelt did.

Other athletes, whose lives may not be immediately threatened by an ailment, have set themselves endurance goals despite some physical limitation. Sometimes the limitation is extreme, as in the case of people confined to a wheelchair or blind or disabled in some other way. Other times the limitations are much less severe. But we are all handicapped in some way; we just vary in the extent to which our handicaps are disabling. When a person with an extreme handicap perseveres against an endurance challenge, those who learn of it are given the message that human will is indomitable. Handicapped athletes seem to benefit in nonathletic areas of their lives by the knowledge that they can achieve substantially in the physical arenas, where they are reputed to have the least ability. Apparently, nonhandicapped people also benefit in the same manner.

Harry Cordellos, who lost his sight as a young man, believes that the only losers in a race are those who don't assemble at the starting line. According to Harry, no matter what your limitations are, preparing for and attempting an endurance test automatically makes you a winner. Thus, compensating for one's physical limitations, whether severe or only minor, has been a powerful incentive for some people to become endurance athletes.

THE HEALTHY ADDICTION

Some athletes joke about being "endurance junkies," claiming an addiction to exercise. Psychiatrist William Glasser has proposed that for many people exercise may cause a healthy addiction. Once people get hooked on exercise, they increase the frequency and duration of their activity much as the drug addict increases dosage. Just as an addict builds tolerance for a drug, the athlete gets into condition and needs more and more exercise to experience the same effects. Long periods of aerobic exercise cause the brain to produce endorphins, substances chemically similar to morphine. Hence, there is an intriguing possibility that there really is a physiological addiction to endurance sport, although the chemical similarity of endorphins to morphine doesn't necessarily mean that they have the same narcotizing effect as that powerful drug. Whatever physiological or psychological processes may be involved, exercise addiction does exist, and endurance athletes may simply be motivated by that addiction. But since the effects of exercise usually are beneficial, this addiction may be, as Glasser says, a healthy one.

NEGATIVE MOTIVATIONS:
THE DARK SIDE OF SPORTS

PERHAPS not all the reasons for participation in demanding endurance athletics are as savory as those depicted in the previous chapter. Promoters of endurance events and some athletes occasionally exploit sports for base or selfish reasons. Also, the addiction to aerobic activity mentioned by psychiatrist William Glasser may not always be so healthy. Could it be that some endurance athletes are following fads, escaping responsibility, ducking interpersonal involvement, or finding an excuse for lack of any other achievement?

EXPLOITATION OF ENDURANCE

The economic distress of the Philippines, which was largely attributable to the concentration of wealth in the hands of dictator Ferdinand Marcos and his regime, has made the trash removal service most Americans take for granted an impossible luxury in that country's capital, Manila. Most of Manila's 1.6 million residents simply burn their garbage in trash cans or holes in the ground, a practice forbidden in most of the world's large cities. The consequence is that Manila is in competition with Los Angeles and Mexico City for the title of "smoggiest city on the planet." There is virtually no way to predict what noxious fumes and toxic gases will be produced by burning garbage that includes plastics and packaging made from exotic petrochemicals. Under these circumstances, it might seem surprising that the running boom hit Manila just as it hit America about a decade earlier. It's difficult to run in the heat and humidity of the tropics, but the smog just adds pulmonary injury to physiological insult. Despite all this, running is now very popular in Manila.

Before Corazon Aquino's victory, Philippine society was polarized. Resistance to the Marcos regime, and outrage over the assassination of Benigno Aquino were the biggest games in town. The running boom is a social phenomenon, and typically each society adapts social movements to its own characteristics. Filipinos were taking sides either for or against the Marcos government. So it should come as no surprise that both sides used endurance athletics for political purposes.

The Marcos government sponsored major footraces and has exploited these as evidence of public support. This was sort of an athletic version of "bread and circuses." Most notable of these government-organized athletic extravaganzas was the Manila International Marathon, whose race director was the deputy minister of sports and whose medals and trophies all were emblazoned with the information that they had been personally donated by Marcos.

Anti-Marcos groups also turned athletic contests into political rallies. The Running Organization for Aquino and the Resignation of Marcos (ROAR) produced weekly 3.7-mile fun runs as a memorial to Aquino. At the height of the fervor over Aquino's martyrdom, ROAR's weekly runs attracted a thousand or more participants. On November 27, 1983, twenty thousand Filipinos jogged or strolled in a fun run that commemorated Aquino's birthday.

In one ROAR event, three hundred runners embarked from Aquino's birthplace, Tarlac, on a 105-mile ultramarathon south to Manila. ROAR called the event the Tarlac-to-Tarmac Run, because they planned for the trek to terminate at the spot on the tarmac of the Manila airport where Aquino died. Along the route, which traversed rural areas of the island of Luzon, many villagers joined the procession. The event's promoters never expected widespread participation in an ultradistance run through the countryside, but by the time they reached Manila the pack of runners had swelled to more than fifty thousand. In an article about ROAR in *City Sport* magazine, Bob Cooper called the Tarlac-to-Tarmac Run "Manila's political Bay-to-Breakers."

The United States has a stable democratic government and a relatively prosperous economy. The level of political fervor is much lower here than in the Philippines. So, apart from occasional participation by individual politicians, American endurance athletics are largely unsullied by politics. But America is an intensely materialist nation. Hence, it should come as no surprise that, in this country, the goals of endurance sport often are distorted for commercial purposes.

Many American endurance events have some level of corporate sponsorship. Naturally, the companies consider their expenditures on an event an investment, and they want to benefit from that in some manner. Sometimes the sponsor takes a benign interest in the contest, providing support and requesting little in return. Other times the companies have been rapacious, as was the case of one corporation that once provided some minor sponsorship for a cross-American bicycle race. The company gave very little money to help the contestants and race organization put on the event, but it spent lavishly on banners and press releases designed to make it appear as though it had underwritten all costs.

Individual American athletes also receive money to endorse or represent products. But it is not always the best athlete who receives the reward. A flair for publicity helps, as was the case of the relatively fast, but certainly not world-class, runner who in the New York City Marathon has worn a waiter's costume and carried a bottle aloft on a tray. In recent races the "waiter" has earned a gratuity. A well-known mineral water company has paid him to conspicuously carry their product on his tray.

Politics and economics are part of the human condition, so it would be naive to expect endurance athletes to remain pristine. Still, these two motivations for participation in endurance sport seem far less lofty than some of the motivations mentioned in the previous chapter.

EXERCISE ADDICTION

All endurance athletes in at least some sense of the phrase are "exercise addicts." Sports are a major part of their lives, and their daily activities. Deprivation of the opportunity to do aerobic exercise brings on withdrawal symptoms. Many endurance athletes claim that after more than two days without exercise they are irritable, jittery, and restless. At best, that addiction might be beneficial, causing them to maintain habits that contribute to psychological and physiological health; at worst the addiction might be physically harmful.

Enthusiasm for endurance sport seems to be a good thing, but a thin line separates enthusiasm from fanaticism. How can that line be drawn? Perhaps theories about compulsive eating can provide a model. When evaluating the dietary habits of the overweight, often a distinction is made between those who eat to live and those who live to eat. Unfortunately, one can't always determine which category is appropriate, so usually people are classified by the results. If they are obese, they may be living to eat.

The same distinction is applicable to exercise addiction. The runner, for example, runs to live; the runaholic lives to run. The person who runs a lot is not necessarily a runaholic; the person for whom running is destructive is a runaholic. If the sport interferes with relationships or prevents productive endeavors, then the runner is very likely a runaholic. As with overeating, looking at the results helps identify the runaholic.

J.T., a thirty-four-year-old runner, had earned a degree in engineering from a prestigious university, in spite of the fact that he had no real interest or drive for that profession. Because he was bright, he had done well in engineering school. When he graduated his real desire was to enter business, for which he lacked any credentials or experience. He followed what he thought was the path of least resistance: worked as an electrical engineer for ten long years, largely because the pay was good and he lacked any other marketable skills.

J.T. hated his work and sought all manner of mental and physical escape from it. As is not uncommon among electrical engineers in California's volatile Silicon Valley, J.T.'s résumé listed nine employers in only ten years. However, unlike many of his peers, J.T. was job hopping to conceal disdain for his occupation, not to seek professional advancement.

J.T. had dabbled in track during college, never showing any great promise as an athlete, but during his unhappy years working as an engineer his running increasingly became an obsession. He used the running as a means to escape thinking about his despised occupation. J.T.'s job performance and professional reputation suffered from his attitude. His projects were completed neither on schedule nor in a satisfactory manner, but by dint of fanatical training he did qualify for the Boston Marathon with a time of 2:47. When his supervisor discovered him out running on one of the many occasions he had called in sick, he got the sack.

This was a catastrophe for J.T. He had always managed to find a new job before his incompetence caught up with him, but now there would be a mark on his record that would be difficult to conceal. He would not be able to get a decent recommendation for a new job.

J.T. sulked for about a week, and then fell back on what he thought he liked best: his running. He formulated a very unrealistic plan. He decided he would win at Boston and thereby show the world he was not a failure. He had always lived from paycheck to paycheck and had saved no money, but when he was fired J.T. received a lump-sum refund of his investment in the company pension plan. He decided he could live on that pittance and train full-time for the next five months. He figured that to win he would need to decrease his marathon time by only thirty minutes or so.

His plan was not very rational, but J.T. set about implementing it with fervor. There were special diets, double and triple split workouts, and ultradistance weeks with speedwork every other day.

The results were predictable: a stress fracture. Recognizing that he had an extreme case on his hands, J.T.'s orthopedist put a cast on his leg so he would not train in defiance of doctor's orders. But the doctor's draconian measures were not good enough. After only a week and a half, J.T. grew weary of his enforced idleness and decided he was all better. Lest he lose any more ground on his training goals, J.T. removed the cast himself and resumed a full schedule of workouts. Later, while in traction at the hospital, J.T. met E.W., a part-time physical therapist, who was herself a recovering runaholic.

At the time J.T. met her, E.W. was a twenty-eight-year-old cocktail waitress with a master's degree in physical therapy and no full-time professional job. An avid runner, she hated hustling drinks for bored, middle-aged businessmen in a sleazy, smoke-filled cocktail lounge. She used to joke that she had become a runner so she would be able to escape her paunchy customers when they made lecherous advances. E.W. had worked her way through school by "cocktailing," as she put it, and she had not yet connected with any full-time opportunities in physical therapy. Besides, when her boyfriend of six years had left her for another woman, she didn't have the energy to look for professional work. In the past she had been very conscious of health and had run for fitness, but at that point in her life running was all she wanted to do. She kept procrastinating about writing a résumé, and just fell into a part-time physical therapy job at the hospital where she had done her internship, where J.T. was recuperating from his injury.

Since her boyfriend had dumped her, E.W. had lost all appetite for food. She had shed 20 pounds as her weekly mileage had simultaneously risen to 130. That brought her 10-kilometer time down to thirty-six minutes, and trophies and other running bric-a-brac began to fill some of the void in her sparsely furnished apartment. When she realized that she was winning races and didn't care, she became a little concerned. But it didn't dawn on her that she might have become anorexic, until she fainted after a week without food. Fortunately, her collapse occurred at the hospital where she worked. While still on intravenous feeding she resolved to seek the help of a psychologist.

Slowly E.W. recuperated. She continued her running, but she also resumed a healthy diet. She began to look for work in her profession. Then she met J.T. at the hospital.

J.T. and E.W. were immediately attracted to one another. J.T. left the hospital after two months, and he and E.W. dated. They eventually married. They borrowed money from friends and family and opened up a fitness spa. E.W. is able to use her professional training in their business, and J.T.'s early desire to be an entrepreneur is fortunately accompanied by a natural aptitude for business. The exercise studio is thriving.

Both of them still run, but J.T. has become more realistic about his athletic goals. He has taken up cycling and swimming as alternative activities that are less likely to cause stress fractures. He does fairly well in local triathlons. Much less manic about footraces, he now pursues running as an avocation that happens to be consistent with his business. E.W. is also realistic about her running: she wins the woman's division of local and regional races with fair regularity. The notoriety this brings has been very helpful to the family business. They often run together, although E.W. takes the sport more seriously than J.T.

Both J.T. and his wife were runaholics. Now J.T. runs moderately, whereas E.W. still puts in heavy mileage. Yet neither one is now a runaholic, because both of them have other meaning in their lives. They run to enhance their lives. Naturally, not all stories end so happily. However, the unhappy ending may be no more common for addicts of endurance sport than for victims of other problems. But perhaps endurance addicts have a better prognosis because the symptom, exercise, is not always harmful.

THE ENDURANCE ATHLETE IN YOU

PART

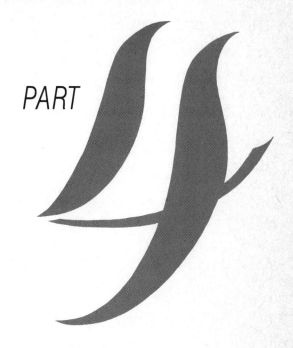

YOU DON'T HAVE TO BE A CHAMPION

NOT ONLY is it unnecessary to become a champion to benefit from endurance sport, in some sense you may already be one. Although the statement that *all* participants are champions can be a dangerously misleading bromide, the major rewards of endurance athletics are intrinsic.

Winning can be defined very broadly. It can include the setting of personal records and the accomplishment of personal goals. Ask somebody who has just completed his or her first triathlon whether it is a victory. As Harry Cordellos said, those who don't assemble at the starting line are the only losers. Still, anybody who has won a competition—or even come close to winning a competition—will tell you just how sweet *real* victory is.

Most of us finish out of the money every time, but that doesn't mean we cannot participate, and it certainly doesn't mean we will derive less benefit from training or competing than the front runners. That insight once came to an acquaintance named Rob in a very difficult manner.

THE HORSE'S ASS TROPHY: WHEN LOSING IS WINNING

In 1964, when Rob was a senior in high school, he began running because he was overweight and out of shape. In those days running was hardly the fad it later became, so Rob always ran alone, wearing a sweatshirt, blue jeans, and Keds all that first winter. At first Rob could barely make it around the block, but he persevered in his solitary workouts, gradually increasing his ability to the point that he could complete a mile and a half round trip, albeit chugging quite wearily up the last hill. Then Rob invested fifteen dollars in a used set of barbells and added a weight workout to his daily fitness activities. Slowly the blubber came off.

Although he became increasingly fit, Rob kept his athletic ambitions extremely modest. Keep in mind that Rob was doing this with

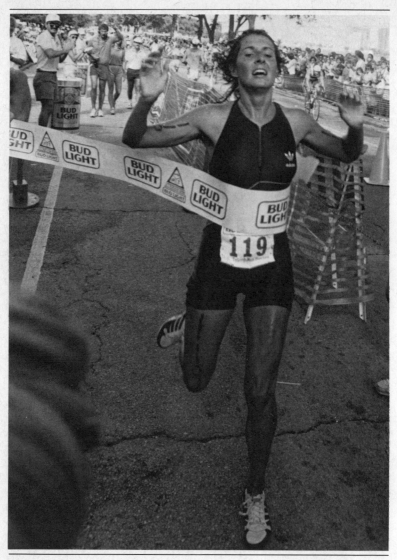

Gaylene Clews apparently knows how sweet winning can be.   COURTESY OF BUD LIGHT USTS

no social support at all, a full decade before the running boom began. The only other runners Rob ever saw were one or two eccentric old men. Even his high school's cross-country and track teams seldom trained on the open roads, and Rob was too close to graduation to consider joining any high school teams. (In fact, he had been cut from the only high school teams for which he had previously tried out.) When Rob first heard about the marathon, a race in which humans are supposed to run 26 miles, he did not believe that such a footrace truly existed. No human could possibly run much more than 2 miles, perhaps 3 at most.

Rob ran purely for fitness. Although he continued running regularly during college, he turned down an invitation to join the college cross-country team. He did not wish to compete, and anyway the collegiate cross-country meets were 5-mile events, and that was a much longer run than he thought possible for himself.

By this point Rob would concede that it was possible for other humans to run farther than 2 miles. But this was only because he encountered living, undeniable evidence of that possibility. Rob's college math professor finished twentieth out of a field of more than one thousand in the 1966 Boston Marathon, with a time of about 2:20.

Because he never competed and never timed his own runs, Rob had no idea whether he was fast or slow. He didn't find out until 1969, after he had graduated from college and was serving as an officer in the navy. He was stationed on a ship in Little Creek, Virginia, and was still running every day. When he was at sea he would run laps around his ship's flight deck. Such fanatical dedication to running was quite an oddity in 1969, so Rob had little recourse but to succumb to peer pressure when his shipmates insisted that he represent them in a 2-mile cross-country race held at their ship's base. Rob initially disliked the idea of competing, but he assumed that if he was in a race he would have to give a full effort and try to win.

Setting his goals so high was a serious mistake. Prior to the running boom, footraces attracted very few contestants. There were only fifteen entrants in that 1969 navy race; fourteen had been high school or college track stars, and then was one other—Rob. Most of the other entrants were members of the navy's elite commando unit, the SEALS, who were training full-time, every day, for hazardous, secret missions in Vietnam. The SEALS were running in excess of 70 miles per week. Then there was Rob, jogging 2 miles or so a day, when conditions permitted, often running less. Yet, on that cloudy day Rob lined up with the track jocks, fully intent upon winning the race. The gun went off and Rob sprinted forward with the best of them. That lasted for about the first 100 yards. Soon Rob was panting and gasping at the back of the pack as the cross-country course took the runners onto the soft sand of the beach. After only a mile Rob could hardly run at all and slowed to a walk.

Then Rob made his worst mistake of the day. Instead of slinking off to lick his wounds and avoid further embarrassment, as any sensible person would have done, Rob decided to finish the race at all costs. The societal injunctions against quitting had been thoroughly drummed into him, and he was concerned that the race officials might be worried about the whereabouts of the fifteenth entrant. Perhaps they would call roll at the finish line, find one sailor missing, and mount a search.

Rob's thinking processes were very muddled at this moment of physical and social distress.

Rob started running again and ultimately crossed the finish line dead last, with a time of a little over fifteen minutes. He wanted to leave the scene of his humiliation, but the race officials prevailed upon him to stay and watch the award ceremonies. Acceding to that request was one more in Rob's long series of mistakes. After the champions, who had completed the race in times of about ten minutes, received their trophies, he finally thought he was free to go. But before he could get away, one more indignity was heaped upon him. The master of ceremonies called him forward and gave him a trophy for finishing the race last. Standing on the trophy's mahogany base was a cast-metal rendition of the hindquarters of a horse. Rob, who had been awarded the horse's ass trophy, faked a good-natured smile as the other runners laughed and cheered.

Inside Rob was crushed. He had entered the race in order to win, not to carry off the booby prize. Worse yet, the award of last-place honors was dutifully reported by the base newspaper, with Rob's name correctly spelled. All of Rob's shipmates read about his defeat. Some had the bad taste to kid Rob about the race. Rob felt compelled to take the jesting good-naturedly, although he ached to say, "Look, you fat jerk, you couldn't run the race at all."

Two years went by, during which time Rob never entered a single race. He had learned his lesson. Remarkably, though, he did continue to run, even when it was dangerous to do so. He enjoyed his running so much that he took foolish risks by running along the back roads at the perimeter of the base where he later served in Vietnam. He might have made a tempting target for a sniper.

Finally, in 1971, friends of Rob's prevailed upon him to enter a 10-mile race in Vallejo, California, where he was then living. At first he was reluctant to enter, but Rob had enjoyed training with his friends so much that he overcame his feelings of shame about the earlier defeat. In the Vallejo race he learned that during the preceding two years the sport of running had undergone a complete metamorphosis. Unlike the earlier race, in which he had been pitted against fourteen track stars, in the Vallejo race there were over two thousand participants. A very small minority of the entrants were champions, some were much slower than Rob, but the vast majority were runners of about his own caliber.

The emphasis had changed, too. Running now seemed to be a mass-participation sport rather than a spectator sport in which thousands might watch a handful of elite athletes display their prowess. What a pleasant surprise for Rob: he had gone away to Vietnam an unskilled devotee of an oddball activity and had returned to a country where his sport was now common and popular. Rob thoroughly enjoyed the race, and it seemed to him that even the last finishers were encouraged rather than taunted by the cheers of the earlier finishers.

During the dozen years after that positive experience with racing, Rob became a regular participant in footraces, triathlons, and bike races. Training for endurance events is now Rob's principal avocation. Rob is not sure why he didn't immediately discard the horse's ass trophy along with his sneakers, but now he is glad he didn't throw away either. He recently has retrieved the statue from the back of the closet and it stands in a place of honor on his mantelpiece.

THERE CAN ONLY BE ONE FIRST PLACE

What is the point of a mass activity in which only one person can be successful? Finisher number one is a winner; finishers two through the last are failures. In the not-too-distant past, the only real role of the failures was to be the supporting cast for the winner in a public spectacle. If one or more of the failures gave the winner a tough race, so much the better; the spectators got a more dramatic show. Naturally, most people were not altruistic enough to take on the role of being one of the losers, and endurance events usually had only a handful of contestants.

Until a decade or so ago, endurance sport was largely a spectator sport, though not nearly as popular as such other spectator sports as football, baseball, and basketball. A probable reason for this is that endurance sport usually lacks the dramatic appeal of team sports and is very difficult to follow. In football, soccer, or baseball all the action is compactly concentrated on one field and each successive play is a brand-new act in the show.

By contrast, endurance events appear boring. Consider a typical cross-country ski race or long-distance swim: "Ready, get set, go!" and they're off; three hours later, at some distant point, here they come, "Hooray!" In between, "Ho hum." Most of the drama of an endurance competition occurs as invisible motivational monologues in the minds of the participants. No wonder endurance sports, such as six-day bike races and six-day runs, which in their time were called "cruelty shows," only enjoyed a brief vogue as spectator sports during the late nineteenth and early twentieth centuries. Then they were completely upstaged by more entertaining sports, such as baseball, football, basketball, and tennis.

Suddenly there appears to be a mass constituency for endurance sport. The explanation for this modern phenomenon probably is participation. True, several million spectators line up on First Avenue and throng the streets of various ethnic neighborhoods in order to *watch* the New York City Marathon. But even this is largely because of personal involvement. Many of those spectators know or are related to one or more of the eighteen thousand participants. It is also true that the telecasts of the Ironman Triathlon and such bicycle events as the Tour de France, Coors Classic, and Race Across AMerica consistently receive high ratings. But here part of the explanation is that the mobile television camera is able to take the spectator along for the ride. The narrator can explain the drama, and television can even peek inside the minds of the contestants by interviewing them before, after, and occasionally during the contest. Given sufficient resources, the camera can always be right where the action is.

Another part of the explanation is that television producers have learned to develop the human interest side of the story, which in reality is what endurance sport is all about. In February 1985, Mike Aisner, the promoter of the Coors Classic Bicycle Race, told an *Ultrasport* interviewer that he thought ABC makes great television out of the Race Across AMerica (RAAM) even though its riders are "the most undynamic personalities on earth." Of course, many people—and athletes—protect their true selves behind bland exteriors. But probing interviewers can break through to the fascinating stories within, particularly when the stress of an endurance event softens the walls hiding the "true" personality. Scenes of Lon Haldeman riding his bike into his hometown of Harvard, Illinois, an unremarkable community of dairy farms, have great emotional impact when placed in the context of a 3,000-mile bike race that has worn away many exterior defenses. The RAAM must be a great challenge to ABC, because the riders are stretched out many miles across the country and rarely are involved in dramatic one-on-one duels. It is the personal struggle that make the RAAM good television; otherwise that race is about as interesting as watching a cow chew the grass in Harvard, Illinois.

The current spectator appeal of endurance sport seems to be based on personal involvement with one or more of the athletes and the thrill of vicariously participating in the race. Endurance athletes report that viewing telecasts of long-distance events inspires them to go out and do the sports they just watched. When the telecast of the Super Bowl finishes, few people have a similar urge to participate in a football scrimmage, even though many of the viewers may have played and enjoyed football in school or elsewhere. The difference is that endurance events are now primarily participation sports rather than spectator sports.

Something changed in modern society to transform spectators into participants. Very likely, heightened awareness of the health benefits of good nutrition and physical fitness is partly responsible for the blossoming of endurance participation. Also, many people now have more leisure time than did their forebears decades ago, and rather than watch television some people fill that time with healthful endurance athletics. One need only venture onto the street or into the public parks to realize that a fitness boom has occurred. Bicyclists, cross-country skiers, lap swimmers, racewalkers, backpackers, mountain climbers, and rowers abound. Single-sport athletics have been followed by the new kid on the block: multisport athletics, which combine two or more of the above sports. As triathlon and biathlon participation burgeons, we are now in the midst of a multisport boom.

Changed attitudes toward competition are also partly responsible for burgeoning participation in endurance sport. Just a decade or so ago football coach Vince Lombardi spoke for most of America when he said, "Winning isn't everything, it's the only thing." In the 1940s it was not uncommon for the front-runners in the Boston Marathon to spill the water bottles that had been set out before the race by their competitors, who were trying to catch them from behind. In the past, sabotaging the competition was just a part of the game, but at least in road racing that attitude has altered dramatically. In 1983, Sister Marion Irvine, a nun and relative newcomer to running who, at fifty-four, qualified for the Olympic marathon trial, expressed the attitude that now prevails. When showing her running trophies to the students at the parochial school where she teaches, Irvine told them, "The goal of competition is self-motivation not victory over others."

Earlier it was asked whether there is any point to a mass activity in which only one person can be successful. The answer is no! Fortunately, the values of athletics have recently been redefined so that all participants who develop and test their endurance can be successful. As that redefinition has occurred, participation in endurance sport has mushroomed.

WOMEN IN ENDURANCE EVENTS

Women's participation in endurance sports has increased dramatically during the last ten years, paralleling the growth in participation by the population in general. In 1974, fewer than 1 million women considered themselves runners; by 1984, that number had increased to 19 million. The rapidly growing sport of triathlon has seen a similar increase in the number of female participants. Recent estimates put the number of triathletes at 1.1 million. About 15 percent (165,000) of those triathletes are women.

Publishers are capitalizing on the fitness boom with so-called fitness magazines aimed at women. More often than not, these magazines are thinly veiled fashion magazines featuring starlets and celebrities sporting the latest in "workout wear": leotards, tights, and legwarmers. They are frequently photographed in suggestive poses, causing the critical reader to wonder to whom these magazines pander. The focus is less on participation in sports than on creating women who fit an updated ideal of beauty.

Another disturbing trend in popular sports publications is the use of "athletic" models who pose for cover shots wearing skintight Lycra suits, or skimpy running shorts in addition to their perfect makeup, coiffures, and more often than not, long, polished fingernails. Those covers sell magazines, yet one wonders about the subtle messages given the consumer of such publications. Wouldn't serious athletes be just as inclined to purchase an issue featuring real athletes such as Joan Benoit, Grete Waitz, Jan Reynolds, or Connie Carpenter-Phinney? Recently, those superstars have graced covers, and with some luck and increased consciousness on the part of sensitive editors and publishers, "real" women will sell more magazines to sports enthusiasts than models ever have.

In a sense, increased awareness has characterized the growth of women's sports since the early seventies. Certainly the women's liberation movement has been a catalyst for women's involvement in sports. The movement addressed the need for women to realize their

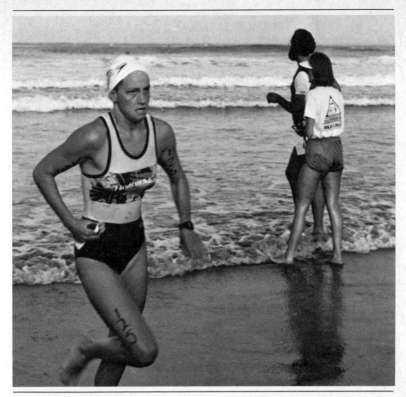

Shannon Delaney emerges from surf at a triathlon in San Diego.   PHOTO BY ALBERT GROSS

absolute equality to men, and consequently, hardly any aspect of American life went unexamined. The growth of the movement and women's awakening consciousness resulted in the dramatic increase in women's participation in sports of all kinds: running, cycling, swimming, horse racing, tennis, golf, and more recently, triathlon, biathlon, mountain climbing, rough-water canoeing, and cross-country skiing.

Prior to the feminist movement, there were notably few female athletes to serve as role models for young women. Such pioneers as "Babe" Didricksen Zaharias, "Fanny" Blankers Koen, Gertrude Ederle, and Sonja Henie paved the way for modern sports heroes like Billie Jean King, Diana Nyad, Grete Waitz, and Joan Benoit. But even with today's role models for young women, endurance sports are still not part of daily life for mainstream society, especially for women.

Women have traditionally been held back in sports by the prevailing opinion that strenuous activity would be injurious to a woman's health. Popular misconceptions have included fear that the female reproductive organs would somehow become dislodged during strenuous activity, that a blow to the breasts could cause cancer, and that

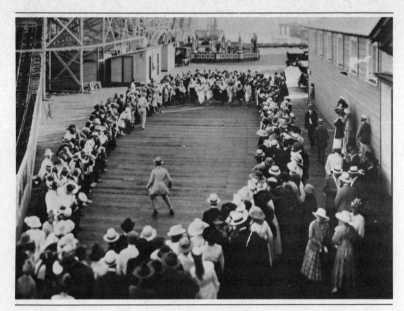

These women wore their Sunday finery to compete in the 1916 "Married Ladies Foot Race" at Santa Monica Pier, California.   COURTESY OF ERNEST MARQUEZ

women were simply too delicate and too fragile to participate. Never mind that women have fared quite well in nomadic societies and that women from cultures such as the Tarahumara Indians of Mexico would run up to 50 miles a day. Women were not encouraged to move around much, except to perform modern household chores.

THE FEMALE ATHLETE'S ADVANTAGES

Female participation in endurance sports has effectively debunked the myths about female physical limitations. Some widely reported studies have suggested that women may be superior to men in some endurance sports due to greater stores of fat. The average highly trained male endurance athlete has 3 to 5 percent fat, the average highly trained female athlete 8 to 12 percent. Some physicians speculate that this fat can be metabolized as fuel during long-distance events. And most marathon runners can attest from observation, if not experience, that fewer women "hit the wall" in a marathon than do men. But researchers continue to debate whether women's additional fat stores are an additional energy source or just plain dead weight.

Unfortunately, there is a tendency to rather carelessly exaggerate the benefits of the female athlete's higher percentage of fat. For instance, it is widely believed that the performance difference between male and female runners decreases as the distance of the event increases. It is thought that at some point the performance curves cross and women allegedly have an advantage. Joan Ullyot, a San Francisco physician and runner, has made that claim in her book *Women's Running*.

In an *Ultrarunning* article that appeared in January 1985, Bernd Heinrich presents statistical evidence that in fact the reverse is true. Looking at world-record running times at various distances, he finds that the longer the distance, the greater the relative gap between men's and women's records. The men's world record time for distances between 400 meters and 2 kilometers are only 11 to 16 percent faster than those for women, whereas the men's times between 50 and 250 kilometers are over 30 percent faster than the women's. A male marathon cyclist, Peter Penseyres, suggests that the slower female times in endurance cycling may be a consequence of the fact that women can't train as much as their male counterparts; the female rider is simply too vulnerable to attack to risk cycling after dark. Female runners suffer similar problems during training, and relatively fewer females run ultradistances than run short distances.

In marathon swimming, however, top female times are frequently better than top male times. Women hold various endurance swimming marks. For instance, Penny Dean holds the world-record time for crossing the English Channel (7:40), and Cindy Nicholas holds the Channel double-crossing record (18:55). During their days of active competition, Gertrude Ederle, Greta Andersen, Florence Chadwick, and Diana Nyad held records for various open-water swims. Perhaps extra body fat truly is a benefit in marathon swimming, where it provides bouyancy and insulation against hypothermia as well as extra fuel.

There are, of course, physical differences other than fat stores that account for the gap in performances. Women, on average, are 4 inches shorter and 29 pounds lighter than men. This smaller size may give women an advantage in sports that involve lifting or propelling one's body (mountain climbing, for example), but it offers little advantage on speed. Women have a lower center of gravity due to a wider pelvis, longer torsos, and concentration of fat on hips and thighs. This may give women a better sense of balance, but it also creates greater knee stress. Narrower shoulders and smaller chests give women less upper-body strength. Men have stronger muscles and greater muscle-building capacity; they also tend to have greater oxygen-carrying capacity than women. One important factor in endurance events is the female's ability to keep cool for a longer period of time than males. Women perspire more efficiently than men and tend to have less difficulty with dehydration.

No amount of medical evidence, however, will soon erase the image of Gabriele Andersen-Schiess, a victim of heat exhaustion, as she entered the Los Angeles Coliseum during the 1984 Olympic marathon. Doubtless, those who are opposed to women's participation in endurance events will use that incident as proof that women risk serious danger to their health. Let's not forget, however, that Alberto Salazar was actually administered last rites by a priest following the 1978 Falmouth Road Race, when he too fell victim to heat exhaustion. Clearly, endurance activity can be dangerous for men and women, not just women.

There are also psychological differences that play an important part in a woman's decision to participate in sports. The process of socialization gives girls and young women very strong messages about femininity and proper behavior for females. Traditionally, playing sports has been seen as an unfeminine activity. Women have been encouraged to be passive, submissive, quiet, and accommodating. Those feminine characteristics are the opposite of the masculine traits of aggression, strength, discipline, independence, and a competitive spirit. Not coincidentally, masculine traits are some of the same qualities essential for success in sports. A woman learns early the social consequences of beating a boyfriend at tennis, of running faster or jumping higher than her brother. Unacceptable behavior is quickly eliminated.

Mary Ann Buxton has endurance credentials that include multiple appearances at the Ironman, the Western States 100-Miler, and the Levi's Ride and Tie. She recalls, "I came from an era in which our mothers taught us that we were to be the supportive people to our

Once exclusively a male domain, crew has become an androgynous sport. PHOTO BY BUDD SYMES

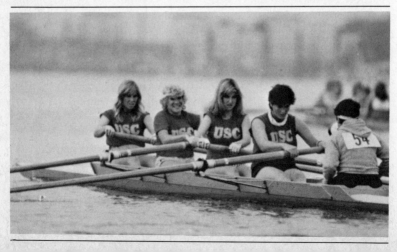

husbands. We weren't to have any particular interest in our own careers or own development or athletics. We were to quit complaining and be the little woman. And that was totally changed as I went through my twenties into my thirties and found that, wait a minute, this is a lot of bunk. There are things that I'm going to do on my own and for myself, and then have a relationship. Men didn't have to go through that. Of course they were going to do things for themselves and develop themselves."

The women's movement has influenced attitudes so that a person of either gender now can express both masculine and feminine traits, leading to what has been termed the "new androgyny." Sharing what is best in both the masculine and feminine roles may be the most humane way to live and certainly will free men and women from the rigidity of their traditional gender stereotypes. When women embrace the aforementioned masculine traits, the result is greater self-esteem, confidence, and feelings of self-control. Studies of women athletes, their sex roles and corresponding achievement, indicate that they score higher than nonathletes on such androgyny indicators as self-esteem and ability to carry through one's plans and set new goals. Men who allow themselves to express such traditionally female attributes as sensitivity and supportiveness increase their ability to cope with the stress of life.

But do females become athletes because they have high self-esteem or do they increase their self-esteem by becoming athletes? We may never know the answer, but one fact is certain: women consistently attribute positive psychological changes to their participation in sport. Female athletes commonly report a sense of mastery, feelings

PHOTO BY BUDD SYMES

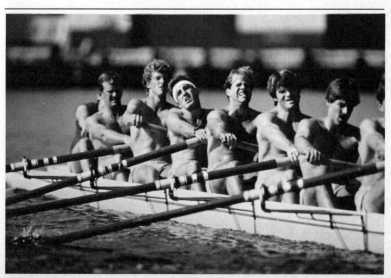

of independence, a newfound pride in accomplishment, and a feeling of conquering the unknown.

A woman who participates in sports makes a statement about her own values and feelings of self-worth. She begins to take control of her body, her time, her level of fitness. Running, cycling, swimming, skiing, and other athletic training requires a woman to make time for herself, away from the demands of home and family. She learns to say no to others and yes to herself, which can upset some traditional relationships. But flexibility, good humor, and a willingness to be creative, especially in the restructuring of conventional roles, will assist a woman to structure her life so as to include sports as a vital component.

The transcendent social importance of successful female participation in endurance sport can hardly be overstated. Examples of female sports champions are an effective rebuttal to arguments that females are physically unsuited to various occupations. In 1984, when Joan Benoit unfurled a huge American flag and took a victory lap around the stadium, she made it seem as if the Olympic marathon had been no more than a stroll in the park for her. With that image in mind, it should be impossible to deny that many women have greater physical ability than many men, even if the average speed, strength, or size of women is less than the average for men.

Many women who have excelled in endurance sports have managed to "have it all": a career in sports, healthy relationships, and even motherhood. Maria Canins, mother of two, won the Coors Classic bicycle race in 1984 at the age of thirty-five; Fordie Madeira, forty-year-old mother of triplets, finished nineteenth in the 1984 U.S. trials for the Olympic marathon team; Bjorg Austrheim-Smith, three-time winner of the women's division of the Western States 100-Miler, is the mother of three; and Shiela Young-Ochowicz, former champion speed skater, came out of retirement from competitive cycling to recapture her world championship crown in track cycling after the birth of her daughter. Runner Valerie Brisco-Hooks, who was forty pounds overweight following the birth of her son, got back into shape with her husband's encouragement and won three gold medals at the 1984 Olympics.

Women actually may have an edge in endurance, because having a child is a formidable biological endurance event. Some physiologists claim that this fact makes women more resistant to the pain and fatigue of long-distance sports.

Some female athletes continue to train during pregnancy. The safety of this for both mother and child has been the subject of some medical debate. A study by sports physician Mona Shangold concluded that the chances of miscarriage (about 15 percent) are no greater or smaller for women who continue to train. Most athletes who maintain their sports regimen during pregnancy reduce the intensity of their workouts and decrease their pace in competition. A few women report that athletic activity has worked for them as an antidote to morning sickness. Researchers do not agree on whether or not exercise during pregnancy deprives the fetus of blood, and on whether infants whose mothers exercised will have normal or low birth weights. Clearly, much more needs to be learned about the effects of exercise on pregnant women and their babies.

Most medical authorities do agree on one thing: expectant mothers should refrain from *increasing* their current level of exertion. Women who have been completely sedentary before will be ill advised to commence a strenuous training program during pregnancy.

THE FEMALE ATHLETE'S MEDICAL PROBLEMS

The physical and psychological benefits for women who participate in sports cannot be denied. But there is at least one fairly common physical disorder in female endurance athletes that is cause for concern. Amenorrhea, the cessation of menstrual periods, is thought to affect up to 43 percent of female athletes. It is common among runners, gymnasts, cyclists, and body builders, all of whom have very low levels of body fat.

Amenorrhea usually occurs when the percentage of body fat drops below 12 percent. It is thought that the body protects itself by ceasing ovulation when it is not prepared to carry a pregnancy. Mother Nature's simple solution to potential problems might be to remove the possibility of pregnancy, although it would be foolhardy to use exercise as a method of birth control.

Amenorrhea may affect future fertility and, because of lowered estrogen levels, *may* contribute to osteoporosis in later life. Female athletes who suddenly cease menstruation (and believe they are not pregnant) should consult with a physician to determine the cause. Amenorrhea may be caused by overtraining, high levels of stress, low body weight, nutritional deficiencies, or hormonal imbalances. It's important, for psychological and physical well-being, to discover the cause.

The findings about the relationship of training and osteoporosis are somewhat contradictory. A regular program of exercise, begun before age thirty-five, may actually prevent osteoporosis. That disease, which involves thinning of the bones, currently affects 6 to 8 million American women. It is common after menopause and is responsible for the so-called "dowager's hump" and the high incidence of broken bones suffered by elderly women. Current research indicates that regular episodes of weight-bearing exercise (running, skiing, skating) can actually increase bone mass and prevent the onset of the disease in one's later years. The catch is that too much exercise may encourage the development of osteoporosis.

Researchers currently believe that women can very safely run from twenty to thirty minutes per day, but that running more than 40 miles per week might change hormone levels enough that the development of osteoporosis would be encouraged. Further research is required, but for now the most prudent prophylactic measure seems to be calcium supplements or adequate calcium in the diet (found in dairy products) and moderation in weight-bearing exercise. The additional benefit of increased calcium in the diet is that the substance is thought to increase endurance by prolonging muscle contractions.

About 55 percent of long-distance runners experience "runner's anemia," primarily because conditioned athletes have an increased need for iron in order for their oxygen-carrying cells to function properly. Since women of childbearing age tend to be low in iron anyway, the problem is exacerbated for endurance athletes. Additional iron in the diet, either from supplements or obtained from food sources (primarily leafy greens and liver), is a good idea. The current Recommended Daily Allowance is 18 milligrams; menstruating athletes may require twice that amount.

Anorexia nervosa, a psychological ailment that affects women far more frequently than men, is an extreme form of self-imposed malnutrition that sometimes afflicts endurance athletes. A 1983 article in *The New England Journal of Medicine* by Dr. Alayne Yates reports that more than 24 percent of anorexic women are intensely involved in athletics. A related disorder, bulimia, in which patients binge and then purge through vomiting or using laxatives, also afflicts some endurance athletes. Bulimia is especially dangerous to athletes because vomiting deprives them of vitamins and other nutrients their bodies desperately need. This ailment also occurs disproportionately among women, perhaps because female status in our society is often perversely linked only to physical attractiveness, and the prevalent standard of beauty is the slender woman. Bulimia and anorexia are difficult to diagnose and treat when they afflict athletes, because for some endurance sports—particularly running and cycling—slim wins. How do you draw the line between dieting to gain a competitive advantage and unhealthy, dysfunctional dieting? The only answer may be the vigilance of the athlete herself and her friends.

THE WOMEN'S MARATHON

Women's athletics have come a long way since the days when women were required to submit health certificates in order to run in a marathon, or those even earlier days when women were not allowed to register at all. The history of the women's marathon is an excellent example of the growth of female participation in endurance sports.

Contrary to common belief, the 1984 Olympics were not the first time that women ran an Olympic marathon. Officially, it was the first time, but the first recorded instance of a woman running a marathon was at the very first Olympic Games in 1896. A woman named Melpomene ran along with the men, finishing unofficially in four and a half hours. It was to be eighty-eight years before the Olympic Games would sanction a women's marathon.

According to popular mythology among runners, Kathrine Switzer was the first woman to run in the Boston Marathon. She was—sort of. In 1967, she obtained a number using the name K. Switzer and did run in the race. During the marathon, race director Jock Semple actually tried to pull her off the course (before her boyfriend intervened). She finished in 4:20 and paved the way for women to be officially accepted in the race in 1972. But she was not the first woman to run the race. In 1966, Roberta Gibb had finished the race in 3:20, though without an official number. She raced again in 1967 and finished in 3:27, but was overlooked because of Switzer's well-publicized encounter with Semple.

But even predating Switzer and Gibb, Marie Louise Ledru completed a marathon in France in 1918. Frances Hayward ran the 54-mile Comrades Marathon and finished an unofficial twenty-ninth out of 68; Violet Percy ran a marathon in England in 1926; Eileen Piper ran up and down Pike's Peak in 1959; and Lyn Carman and Merry Lepper raced unofficially in a Southern California marathon in 1963. The women were already off and running when Switzer came along. Trouble was, nobody knew it.

Switzer's appearance at Boston inspired other women, and they decided to run in the race, officially or not. In 1968 and 1969, two women finished; in 1970, five women completed the race; and in 1971, three women raced. By 1972, women marathoners had won several moral victories of which they could be proud; the Amateur Athletics Union (AAU) finally recognized and allowed women's participation in marathon racing, the Boston Marathon allowed women to race, and the Olympic officials decided to add the women's 1,500-meter run to the upcoming Games.

In 1971, women served notice that not only did they want to race, they wanted to race fast. Beth Bonner became the first woman to run the marathon in under three hours, winning the New York City race in 2:55.22. Nina Kucsick finished that race second, in 2:56.04. By 1974, the first U.S. AAU National Marathon Championship for women was held in San Mateo, California, attracting fifty-seven runners (forty-four finished, led by Judy Ikenberry in 2:55.17). In September of the same year, the first women's international marathon was held in Waldniel, West Germany. Marathoning was on its way to becoming an international sport for women as well as men.

In 1978, Avon hosted its first International Marathon in Atlanta, Georgia, a race that attracted top talent from nine countries. Avon was to become a leading force behind the movement to include the women's marathon in the Olympic Games. Also in 1978, Grete Waitz appeared on the scene in New York and won her first marathon in a world record time of 2:32.30. She was to repeat her win in 1979 with a 2:27.33, in 1980 with a 2:25.41, and in 1982, 1983, 1984, and 1985. New York became the favorite race for the Norwegian runner, who was treated like the fair-haired queen of the road each October.

Women's marathon times continued to fall, and there were more and more women's international road races held in venues such as Tokyo, London, New York, Los Angeles, Athens, and Waldniel. The number of female participants continued to increase, until an impressive turnout of more than forty-three hundred women ran at the New York 10-Kilometer Mini-Marathon in 1978. No longer could the AAU (now TAC, The Athletics Congress) claim that not enough women were participating in the sport, that distance running was too dangerous, or that not enough countries would support the event in the Olympics. Finally yielding to growing pressure, the International Olympic Committee announced in 1981 that the 1984 Olympic Games would include a women's marathon race. It was a sweet victory for such pioneers as Kathrine Switzer, Grete Waitz, Nina Kucsick, Jacqueline Hansen, and Joan Ullyot.

Although the marathon was included, the 5,000- and 10,000-meter races have still not been added to the Olympic agenda for women, despite a lawsuit filed by female athletes who wanted to see those events included in the 1984 Games. There seems to be no doubt that continued pressure and lobbying will eventually lead to inclusion of these events, probably for the 1988 Games in Seoul.

In some sports other than running, women are still overlooked, as happened in the 1984 Race Across AMerica. Though four women entered that race, they were not given a separate division and hence all four were officially disqualified according to a rule that drops any-

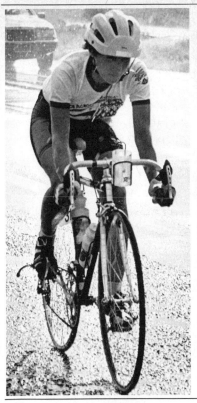
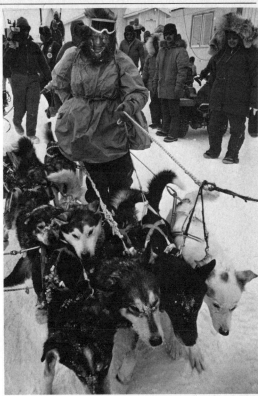

LEFT: *Shelby Hayden-Clifton toughing it out during a Race Across AMerica rainstorm.* PHOTO BY DAVE NELSON

RIGHT: *Libby Riddles and her victorious Iditarod team in Koyuk, Alaska.* PHOTO BY GREG ANDERSON

body who falls thirty-six hours behind the leader. Three of the women actually finished, although no race official was present at the Atlantic City pier to declare a winner when Shelby-Hayden Clifton and Pat Hines culminated a 3,000-mile race with a neck-and-neck sprint.

To their credit, the RAAM promoters responded to public criticism by making the female race a separate event the next year. Susan Notaragello-Haldeman thereby became the first official female finisher, when she won the women's division race of the 1985 RAAM.

WOMEN IN THE WINNER'S CIRCLE

The accomplishments of female athletes continue to astonish and amaze. In 1985 Libby Riddles became the first woman to ever win the 1,100-mile Iditarod Trail Dog Sled Race, collecting a $50,000 check for her eighteen-day trek through Alaska's wilderness from Anchorage to Nome. Jan Reynolds, who has been the subject of increased media attention, sees endurance sports as a way of life. She has completed the Everest Great Circle (climbing around the mountain rather than up it), competes in the Mountain Man Triathlon, and finished fourteenth in the 1984 Biathlon World Championships. (Nordic biathlon is a martial sport that involves cross-country skiing and target shooting with a rifle.)

Diana Nyad, a former endurance swimmer who set a world record when she swam from Florida to Cuba, a distance of 89 miles, is frequently seen as a sports commentator and host on ABC-TV. Her annual pilgrimage with the bicyclists of the Race Across AMerica is the highlight of her year. Discerning viewers will recognize her ability to empathize with other endurance athletes who are pushing the limits.

The world's record for the women's marathon continues to fall, as it did in 1985, when Norway's Ingrid Kristiansen won the London Marathon in 2:21.06. Kristiansen managed to pocket a cool $75,000 purse for her win, which proves that women are moving into their rightful place as athletes who deserve to be compensated for their performances, sacrifices, and training, just as men are.

Athletic women will know that the sporting world is truly equal when books of this sort no longer contain chapters dealing with women, when magazines no longer feature a special women's section, and when it is realized that the phrase "female athlete" is redundant.

CHAPTER ▐▌▐▌▐▌▐ ■ ▶14

GETTING INVOLVED

*T*HIS IS the only "how-to" chapter in the entire book. If you are wondering how to get involved in endurance sport, this chapter will offer some help.

DECIDING

Pursuing endurance sport involves a substantial personal commitment, usually for a period of years. There may be some sacrifice involved. If the stories in this book have inspired you to become an endurance athlete, you ought to consider what you are willing to give up to achieve your goal. Those potential costs should be carefully weighed against what you stand to gain.

One particular athlete, Ken, has done well in his age group in the Ironman Triathlon. He would like, at least once, to win the men's 55–59 age division of that race. He is aware that achieving this ambition is no trivial project; the "old farts"—as many of his peers in the Ironman call themselves—are a highly competitive group. Current times for the first finisher of Ken's division rival those of the overall winner in the early Ironman races. To win his division, Ken will have to train diligently for at least the next year. Then illness or injury might prevent accomplishment of his goal, as happened once when dehydration (helped along by a recent bout of flu) forced him to quit at mile 90 of the bike portion—while in first place for his division.

The training appears to be the least of the sacrifices that Ken has made for his goal. In fact, he enjoys the workouts. Ken was at a point in his life that allowed him to retire from his job as a teacher in order to move to the Big Island of Hawaii to train full-time. That change in his life was welcome, but he also had to give up his beloved Southern California cottage perched on a picturesque cliff by the Pacific Ocean.

What does Ken stand to gain? Precious little of a tangible nature. Perhaps a trophy, but no million-dollar contract with a professional team. The rewards for his effort are all intrinsic. The world will not

215

notice if he accomplishes his goal, but *he* will know. And win or lose, his wife, friends, and two sons (also Ironmen) will applaud. Certainly most people would applaud, although they themselves might not accept the steep trade he is making to pursue his endurance dream.

Virtually anybody who is in reasonably good health *could* become an endurance athlete. However, that doesn't mean that you should make the required sacrifices. Only you can decide, but two factors can help you make that decision. First, the decision is always revocable. Each day's training is a brand-new decision about endurance sport, and at any time you can desert the sport to resume the activities you may have temporarily abandoned. (Ken's teaching credentials will still be valid if he decides to resume his previous occupation.) Second, there are varying levels of commitment. Many—perhaps most—endurance athletes regard their sport as an avocation. Most endurance athletes work full-time at conventional occupations and still find time for regular training. Many activities can fit in one day, and many people create time for family, profession, and endurance sport, as well as other hobbies and vices.

The decision to pursue endurance sport also can be made incrementally. That is, you can escalate the extent of your commitment: for instance, graduating from 10-kilometer footraces to marathons and from marathons to ultramarathons. Actually, the weakness of human flesh practically requires that the decision be made incrementally. Overtraining and excessive ambition have injured many novices. So, before you start rowing across the Atlantic, see if you can make it across the local pond. You will be able to decide more intelligently about the advisability and desirability of grandiose endurance ambitions once you have met and overcome smaller challenges. Using the incremental approach to endurance may take the decision out of your hands because, in the process of escalating, you will automatically discover where your abilities and preferences lie.

Suppose you set your sights on joining a future Everest expedition. Since no serious expedition would even consider taking a novice along, you would have a long apprenticeship ahead of you. Perhaps you would learn basic rock climbing, ice climbing, and general mountaineering techniques. Let us say you build your cardiovascular capacity by running and pursuing other aerobic sports. Then you might climb the glacier of Mount Rainier in the company of experienced guides, only to discover that you become wretchedly sick from breathing the thin air at the 14,408-foot summit of that mountain. (Humans vary in their abilities to acclimatize to high altitude.) Hence, you might be wise to rule out the grand peaks of the Himalayas forever. Everest is more than twice as high as Rainier, and you must survive for weeks at over

20,000 feet, often without artificial oxygen, to get near its summit. Does that mean you can't still enjoy hiking or rock climbing at lower altitudes? Might you not still benefit physically and psychologically from climbing 6,293-foot Mount Washington in New Hampshire, or any number of lesser mountains? Also, should an unpleasant experience on Mount Rainier preclude other endurance sports?

The very nature of endurance sports means that you can't excel at more than a few of them at any one time. Multifitness and cross-training are beneficial, and factors such as aerobic capacity can serve you in several sports simultaneously. However, there are specific muscles that must be trained for any given sport—i.e., cross-country skiing muscles are different from swimming muscles—and there are limits to the time available for training. Endurance athletes probably should pursue only a few major goals at one time.

If you have made the decision to pursue an endurance sport, you would be wise to set and meet performance goals. To make your athletic goals effective motivators and guides for behavior, you should make them as concrete as possible.

Experts on goal setting tell us that concrete goals have tangible bench marks of achievement. Thus, the goals must refer to measurable behaviors rather than states of being: "I will run three miles," instead of "I will become a runner." Beyond that, concrete goals have deadlines and specific standards of accomplishment. Thus the vague goal "I'm going to be a good triathlete" will probably not inspire performance as effectively as a specific goal: "I will complete the Atlanta U.S. Triathlon Series race this season in a time under two hours and fifteen minutes."

At ten years old Penny Dean had set herself the formidable goal of swimming across the English Channel. As she developed into a fine endurance swimmer over the ensuing thirteen years she chose some important subgoals. She decided that she wanted to set a new female record for the Channel. Then she decided that she wanted to set the overall Channel record, for both men and women. Finally, she decided that she wanted to break the seemingly impossible eight-hour barrier.

As the day for her attempt approached, Dean wanted to motivate herself to train specifically for her goals. She says she accomplished that by using self-hypnosis. She programmed herself to be reminded of her goal every time she saw a red dot. She pasted red dots on her luggage and various other personal items, and every time she saw the red taillights of an automobile or a red traffic signal she was reminded of her goal. She says the constant reminder of her goals caused her to redouble her training efforts. If success is any proof, it seems that her somewhat obsessive motivational approach works. Dean achieved all her goals when she crossed the Channel in seven hours and forty minutes.

You can make your goals as ambitious or modest as you wish, but unless they are clearly defined they will scarcely help you get involved at all. In fact, experts on goal setting generally agree that the most effective goals are those that stretch expectations just a little bit, but are not so ambitious that they are overwhelming. Unrealistically ambitious goals ultimately discourage performance improvement because they doom you to failure. No matter what you say your goal is, you will never run a marathon in one hour.

ASSESSING POTENTIAL

During the late 1960s the so-called human potential movement promoted the idea that all things are possible for all people. In many quarters, that philosophy has survived intact to this day. What a cruel deception! If all people can accomplish all things, then anybody who has not yet accomplished some particular goal must be a shiftless failure. Thus, one would be justified in blaming *all* victims of such social calamities as poverty for their own fate. The haves always are more prone to say "Any child can grow up to be president" than are the have-nots. Belief in unlimited potential denies that such obvious individual differences as innate talent and opportunity exist.

Disregarding physical limitations, however, all people are probably capable of accomplishing a little bit more than they have already. Very likely that is the case for athletics. But before your unbridled ambition condemns you to inevitable failure, you should assess your potential in a realistic manner.

How do you assess your potential for a particular endurance sport? Here is a four-step procedure:

1. First consider how well you have done in that sport in the past. Previous performance is the best forecaster of future performance. An active participant in a sport will have plenty of information on which to base an assessment. Take, for example, running. Suppose you know that your marathon time improves markedly as a result of interval training and you also know that running intervals does not injure you. Then the chances are that doing more speedwork will further improve your performance. If you have not pursued a particular sport since your youth, then your performance during those earlier years might provide a clue to your present potential. For the complete neophyte, looking at performance in activities that use similar groups of muscles may help assess potential. For

instance, knowing how strongly you bicycle can help you predict how fast a speed skater you might be.

2. Give the sport a fair trial. Your improvement is the most important factor in judging your potential in a sport. Thus, a fair trial is generally more than one or two attempts. You have to get past the awkward beginner stage before an assessment is possible.

3. Get an expert opinion. Let a coach or some other devotee of the sport observe your performance and give you some feedback.

4. Then, and only then, draw some conclusions about how far you may go with your ultimate goals for the sport. But be willing to revise your assessment on the basis of future triumphs or disappointments.

HOW TO TRAIN

Every sport has unique characteristics that dictate which training approaches will work. Endurance sports, however, are similar enough to justify some generalizations. All endurance sports require cardiovascular fitness, strong muscles, and skillful, efficient movement.

Study Your Sport

The first step for the beginning endurance athlete is to gather information. Learn as much as you can about your sport. Learn where, when, and how it is done. Learn the hazards. Learn the potential rewards.

Where do you obtain such information? Join a club. You can locate a sports club by asking at a store or facility that specializes in your sport. The folks at a good bike shop can tell you about local cycling teams, and those at a mountaineering shop will know about cross-country ski clubs and rock-climbing organizations. Similarly, the lifeguard at the local pool or beach may be able to refer you to a masters swimming program. Athletic club representatives are often at track meets, road races, bicycle races, and swim meets. Members of clubs often wear their organizations' insignia on their clothing while training or competing, and they would probably be glad to tell you how to join.

If you can't locate a local team, you might inquire at a national organization for the sport. For instance, the U.S. Ski Association (1750 East Boulder Street, Colorado Springs, Colorado 80909) can provide information about local Nordic ski clubs. Information about local running clubs is available from the Road Runners Club of America, 8811 Edgehill Drive, Huntsville, Alabama 35802. Local cycling clubs affiliated with the United States Cycling Federation can be located by inquiring at USCF, 1750 East Boulder Street, Colorado Springs, Colorado 80909. Similar information about swimming clubs is available from United States Swimming, 1750 East Boulder Street, Colorado Springs, Colorado 80909.

Don't overlook publications either. Many sports have associations that publish regular magazines or newsletters. For instance, the U.S. Rowing Association publishes *Rowing U.S.A.* Commercial magazines, such as *The Runner, Runner's World, Triathlon,* and *Winning: Bicycle Racing Illustrated,* cover their respective sports. *Ultrasport,* and *Outside* cover endurance sport in general. The recommended readings and the periodicals listed at the conclusion of this book offer a wealth of information about endurance sports.

After you've done some reading on endurance sport, remember: there is no substitute for experience. No amount of vicarious participation can tell you what mile 24 of the footrace in the Ironman feels like. You have to discover that for yourself.

Obtain the Tools of the Trade

Armed with a little knowledge, the next step is to begin accumulating equipment. Endurance sports vary greatly in both the amount and cost of the equipment required. Running, for instance, has comparatively low equipment costs. The most expensive running shoes won't set you back much more than $150, and the norm is under $75. Usually the choice of shoes is dictated more by personal requirements than by any general superiority of the more costly models; more money won't necessarily buy more comfort. Similarly, swimming usually requires very little equipment beyond goggles and a swimsuit. Of course, pool usage fees can add up to a good deal more. On the other hand, cyclists, cross-country skiers, and rowers usually must invest a great deal of money in athletic equipment, and in those sports better equipment sometimes does make life easier.

There is one important factor to consider when shopping for athletic equipment. Whether you choose a penny pincher's sport or a plutocrat's, you can't buy athletic performance. How diligently you train will influence your performance much more than how much the sporting-goods store adds to your credit card bill.

At least initially, it usually is wise to rent or borrow equipment for high-ticket sports such as cross-country skiing. The flexibility of rentals will allow you to try numerous options. There is a fairly robust market for secondhand equipment, particularly in such sports as bicycling and skiing. Publications about the sport often list used equipment in classified ads; clubs often sponsor swap meets; and some stores take trade-ins and deal in secondhand equipment. During the second stage of your career in an endurance sport, you can continue to experiment by participating actively in that secondhand market. Once you are truly informed about equipment, you can trade up to new and higher-quality bicycles, skis, and rowing shells, selling your old equipment in that same used-equipment marketplace.

Design a Training Schedule

Training schedules are like toothbrushes: we all should use them, but we'd probably be better off if we didn't share them. You, or perhaps you and your coach, should design your own unique training plan. Still, there are some general guidelines about how to train and how much to train that can be mentioned here.

Endurance sports require cardiovascular conditioning, as well as strength and skill. Unlike such sports as tennis, racquetball, or baseball, you can't participate in endurance sports sporadically. Even if your tennis racket hangs in the closet untouched for years, you can still take it out and play a few sloppy sets. But it is extremely difficult and dangerous to run a marathon or do a century ride (100 miles) on a bicycle if you have neglected your cardiovascular training. Regularity and consistency of training are essential if you want to participate safely and skillfully in endurance sports. Unlike skill sports such as tennis or bowling, no amount of natural talent can make up for the failure to train for endurance sports.

It is virtually impossible to perform as an endurance athlete on fewer than three workouts per week, and a schedule of daily workouts (with a rest day every week or two) seems to work best. In fact, serious endurance athletes often do split workouts, practicing their sport or related sports two or more times per day.

Specifics about how much to train vary by sport, goals, and individual background. Some examples might help you decide what you need to do in order to meet your goals. In the April 1984 issue of *Ultrarunning,* Bill Schultz published the results of a training survey answered by twenty-one of the twenty-seven runners who had entered a forty-eight-hour race. For that group of ultramarathoners, the long-term training base varied from a low of just 38 miles per week to a high of 112 miles per week. Most of the runners who responded to Schultz's survey increased their mileage during the two months prior to the forty-eight-hour event, just as most runners would do for a marathon. During the final two months, average weekly mileage ranged between 44 miles and 122 miles for those twenty-one runners.

For triathlons, your individual physiology and goals should determine how much to train. It's risky to recommend specific training requirements, but it is possible to suggest minimums that might be sufficient preparation for a long and a short triathlon. For a short event (1-mile swim, 25-mile bike, and 6-mile run) you would be wise to start your training at least three months prior to the event, and you could probably get by with about twelve hours training per week, including weekly splits of 5 miles (8,800 yards) swimming, 75 miles bicycling, and 25 miles running. When asked what would be minimally satisfactory for an Ironman-length event, John Howard, who won the 1981 Ironman, said, "Assuming you have a good, strong background as a runner or cyclist, you probably could get by on 250 miles of bicycling, 40 miles of running, and 20,000 yards [11.36 miles] of swimming per week. You probably should start that program at least six months before the event and peak on the day of the race. Of course, to do well in the race you'll have to do a lot more work than that."

When training for triathlons it makes good sense to evenly distribute the workouts across the week, usually doing no more than two of the sports on any given day.

Penny Dean has written a brief training manual called *How to Swim a Marathon*.* For a swim of the 21-mile Catalina Channel, Dean recommends that swimmers start at least a year in advance and train six days per week, alternating hard and easy days. She emphasizes that building speed is as important as building endurance, because you need to be able to make progress against rapid tides and currents. The speed is built by swimming sets of ten sprints of 100 yards in length, in a pool or the ocean. The swimmer should rest five to thirty seconds between each 100-yard sprint. Repeat the sets three to ten times per workout. To counteract boredom, vary the workout by changing the number of sprints and distance. For instance, five 200-yard sprints is roughly equivalent to ten sprints at 100 yards.

During the one-year preparation period, the swimmer should also do one long, continuous practice swim each month, gradually increasing the distance from 2 miles the first month to 17 miles the eleventh month. The swimmer should taper down during the month of the actual swim. For an event shorter than the 21-mile Catalina Channel swim— let's say a 10-mile lake swim—the training can be scaled down proportionately.

Endurance athletics is not a trivial commitment. Yet quality of training is often as important as quantity, and it is distinctly possible to overtrain, injuring muscles, joints, tendons, and other assorted body

How to Swim a Marathon is available from United States Swimming, 1750 East Boulder Street, Colorado Springs, Colorado 80909. As of the summer of 1985, the charge is $4.00 plus postage.

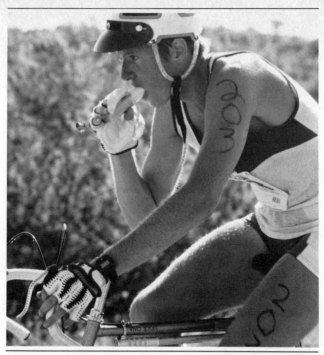

Unlike other athletes, triathletes such as Barry Rick must train to be comfortable eating during long-course events.
PHOTO BY BUDD SYMES

parts. Although distance competitors must get their occasional long workouts to accustom their bodies to long periods of exertion, regular moderate workouts are generally more beneficial than less frequent long ones. Thus, an athlete who swims a mile or so six days per week will be better trained for endurance swimming than someone who just swims 10 miles every Saturday.

The necessity for regular workouts requires that you be realistic about your training schedule, weighing your athletic goals against your other time constraints. If other responsibilities will not permit scheduling the amount of training you need during prime time, then you may need to reassess your goals. Of course, every case is unique, but it is difficult to stick to training schedules that require workouts at four in the morning. You may be disciplined enough to be up that early, but if you don't compensate by retiring early, sleep deprivation will ultimately stop you. As you increase training, the problem gets worse because longer workouts seem to increase sleep requirements.

Still, it is possible to fit quality training time into a variety of different schedules and life-styles. For instance, Mary Ann Buxton trained for ultramarathons, the Ironman Triathlon, and the Levi's Ride

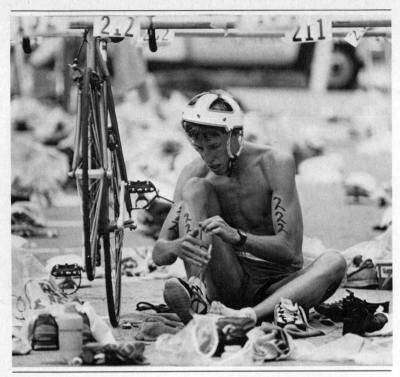

*Be sure to train for rapid transitions between segments
of a triathlon. Chris Hinshaw quickly prepares to run.*
COURTESY OF BUD LIGHT USTS

and Tie while employed full-time as a corporate executive for Levi Strauss and also, for part of that time, was enrolled in a master's degree program. She trained early in the morning, during her lunch hours, and after work. Often she was able to economize on time by doing two things at once. She accomplished many of her personal errands at nearby business establishments during her lunchtime run, and she did much of the required reading for her courses while she pedaled an indoor exercycle. By using note cards that she carried with her, Mary was able to memorize facts for some courses while she ran. Naturally, it helped that her husband, Bart, is also an endurance athlete and shared his wife's fanatical dedication to athletic training.

Many people use their commuting time to get daily workouts. If you can solve such logistical problems as showering and changing clothes, you may be able to bicycle, run, cross-country ski, or even row to and from work.

That's right. It is even possible to row to work, and you don't have to be employed as a lifeguard either. In Chicago, Michael Marty, an office worker, paddles a 19-foot kayak to work. He leaves the boat at a Chicago River pier and hoofs it the remaining mile to his office.

From his craft, which he paddles at a cadence of 30 strokes per minute, he can watch the traffic jam on nearby streets. No problems dodging aggressive motorists on the freeway, although he still has to contend with some of Lake Michigan's commercial boat traffic. Chicago is a busy port.

You may fear that training during rush hour will not permit you to attain excellence in your sport. Peter Penseyres, a supervising engineer at Southern California Edison's San Onofre Nuclear Power Plant, rides his bike to work every day—rain or shine, hot or cold— 56 miles round trip. There are some gnarly hills between the plant and his house in rural Fallbrook, California. He works eight hours a day, five days a week, has a happy marriage and a fourteen-year-old daughter, who doesn't seem neglected. But still he finds time to pursue endurance sport. And he is a high achiever athletically as well as professionally. Squeezing in a substantial part of his training while commuting, Penseyres won the 1985 Race Across AMerica (RAAM), setting a record of nine days, thirteen hours, thirteen minutes for the 3,047-mile transcontinental ride. Not bad for your average work-a-daddy.

The ride to and from work was not enough to win, but the commuting gave Penseyres a minimum training base of five 56-mile days per week. When he peaked his training for the RAAM, he added extra mileage each day and a 400-mile training ride each weekend. His wife met him after work on Friday with a van to support the long ride, and he rode nonstop through Friday night and all day Saturday until he had covered 400 miles. The long ride accustomed him to the sleep deprivation required by the RAAM. In all, he rode between 800 and 1,000 miles per week each of the last ten weeks of his training, and he never missed an hour of work to do so.

Penseyres claims that working while he trained was an advantage over those RAAM competitors who trained full-time. He had other interests to keep his life entertaining, and the schedule constraints made it easier for him to "decide" whether or not to train. When the time came to do it he had to respond immediately, regardless of his current morale. If he did otherwise he would not have been able to recapture the opportunity.

One nice feature of endurance athletics is the usefulness of cross-training. All the endurance sports require cardiovascular fitness, and training for any of them will build this type of fitness. Thus, a runner can make rapid progress in cycling or cross-country skiing. Also, conditioning for any of these sports can be maintained during the off-season by workouts in one of the other sports. Unfortunately, that fact also presents a potential hazard. If you have the requisite endurance, it's easy to overdo it—straining untrained tendons and muscles in a sport you haven't practiced much. For instance, one runner took up swimming as part of a program to become a triathlete, swam too far the first few workouts, and was sidelined by biceps tendinitis. The running had built enough endurance to permit him to injure the under-developed upper body. Still, cross-training effects make it possible to schedule a lot more endurance training than the durability of one set of otherwise overused muscles would allow.

Find Mentors and Training Buddies

If you are at all serious about a sport, the time will come when you need coaching. Not that you can't learn an awful lot from personal experience and reading about endurance sports. It's just that an objective, well-informed third party can see your good and bad habits as no self-observation could.

A knowledgeable coach will of course be able to teach you specific skills of your sport. He or she can help you correct mistakes, urge you to try new techniques, and monitor your progress. A coach can also help you muster the self-discipline necessary to adhere to an ambitious training schedule. There is nothing like knowing that your coach will ask for a report to inspire conscientious training on days that you feel lazy. Accountability works wonders.

One of the positive features of endurance sport is that you can do it alone. You don't have to coordinate schedules with other people, as you do with court sports or team sports, so you can get your workout at a time that suits you or in a town where you don't know anybody. If you need some time for introspection or solitude, a long bike ride in the country or paddling alone in your kayak will serve you well. Yet endurance sports also permit pleasurable interaction with training buddies.

Triathlete Dave Scott, who has won the Ironman four times, usually trains alone because he chooses to live in Davis, California—many miles north of San Diego, where the majority of his serious competitors reside. Many San Diego triathletes train together, and at one point many of the more talented ones—Scott and Jeff Tinley, Mark Allen, Scott Molina, Kathleen McCartney, and John Howard—were all lavishly sponsored by the now-defunct Team JDavid. (Team JDavid came to an abrupt end when the securities empire of Jerry David Dominelli crumbled amidst charges of fraud and violations of federal law.)

Although Dave Scott often trains alone, he denies that one must become a recluse to be successful at endurance sport. He claims his reputation as a solitary athlete is greatly exaggerated; he does train with other people when possible. "In fact," he says, "I'm very people oriented. I've never been a loner. That reputation is caused by geography not choice. It's 11:00 A.M., who can I call up to go running? There isn't an endless supply of training partners in a small town like Davis." Still, some sports commentators continue to perpetuate the myth that endurance athletes concentrate best on their training when they are reclusive.

For what it is worth, it seems that endurance sport gives you great flexibility on the matter of social versus solitary training. The nature of endurance sport allows you to train alone when circumstances or preference requires it. At other times endurance training can be a crucial shared activity in a relationship. Many people train with spouses, siblings, parents, or friends. The training time spent together seems to help to cement the relationship.

Build Toward Your Athletic Goals

Endurance is built slowly and carefully. If you want to make rapid progress, you would be wise to seek sports or activities other than those described in this book. For endurance sports you must first build a base, both in general aerobic fitness and in the specific skills and strength requirements of your particular sport. You must make sure you can walk before you run.

If you are patient, building slowly and persevering, results will come. Your body will change in slow, imperceptible increments if you train regularly. The cardiovascular training effects will occur, and your musculature will change in the direction of the physique characteristic of your sport. Rowers and swimmers will appear beefier in the upper body; cyclists and runners will shift much of their bulk to south of the equator. Perhaps the mirror won't show such gradual changes, but looking at an old photo, or a reunion with somebody who hasn't seen you for a while, will inform you that you have changed.

Compete on Occasion

During the long months of training, the changes in your level of conditioning will be subtle. Unless you compulsively keep records during training, short-term skill fluctuations will be difficult to notice. But when you compete, with somebody else acting as timekeeper, you get very objective evaluations of your current ability.

There are other reasons to compete. Competitions have a social aspect; they are an opportunity to meet or renew acquaintances with people who share your interest in the sport. Competitive events give you a goal for your training. They expose you to new techniques, equipment, and ideas. They are usually fun, if you have realistic expectations. Competition also serves a valuable purpose by publicizing

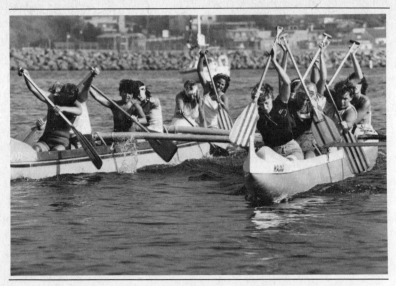

The women of the Marina del Rey, California, Outrigger Canoe Club get their workouts on the group plan.
PHOTO BY BUDD SYMES

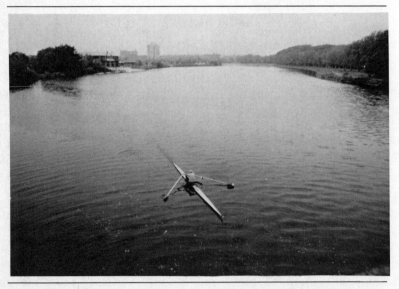

A sculler on the Charles River getting his exercise alone.
PHOTO BY BUDD SYMES

your sport to the community at large; it's much easier to find equipment, training buddies, and tolerance of your sport if nonparticipants have a clearer notion of what is involved in it.

How do you locate the competitive meets? The same resources that provide training information can inform you of opportunities to compete: publications, other athletes, clubs, and stores. Occasionally an event will be so widely publicized in the general-circulation media that you will have difficulty not learning of it in advance. Athletes who do not live near a large metropolitan area may need to travel in order to compete as frequently as they wish.

If you are willing to help promote or produce competitions either on your own or under the auspices of a club, then you can directly influence the accessibility of competition. The six-day race is a good example. That sport was defunct until ultradistance runner Don Choi organized the first modern six-day race in San Francisco. Now that sport is experiencing a renaissance. Another example is the ride and tie, which didn't exist until Bud Johns invented it as a promotional event for his employers, Levi Strauss.

A FINAL WORD ON GETTING INVOLVED

Participation in endurance sport is not suited for everybody, but it can be a metaphor of anybody's personal struggle. Endurance sport can be beneficial to just about anybody who approaches it correctly. What is the "correct" approach? Probably it's the one that lets you get what you want from the sport. If distance rowing or cycling or cross-country skiing or running or swimming or some other endurance activity causes physical and psychological effects you desire, then you have approached the sport correctly. Take what you wish from the advice here, but adapt it to your idiosyncratic needs. Most of all, enjoy!

TRAINING AND RELATIONSHIPS

"I WAS A triathlon widow," laments Peggy Grider in the March 1985 issue of *Triathlon* magazine. Her story is entertaining, though also stereotypical and predictable. She was a nonathlete, whose only exercise was "running up the staircase every night to bed." Suddenly, her husband, LeRoy, who only had played a couple of racquetball games each week, became a man obsessed with his training for the Lancaster County (Pennsylvania) YMCA Triathlon, which included a 1.2-mile swim, a 25-mile bike race, and a 9.3-mile run. With tongue in cheek, she described the accommodations she made to her husband's new sport, which required buying an expensive bicycle and one to three hours per day of rigorous multisport training. She worried about his safety and seemed to resent the time he spent training, but liked the improvement in physical health and self-esteem that she saw in him. At the end of the article we learn that she has begun to train too.

One professional bicycle road racer believes that withdrawal of support for his athletic endeavors paralleled the breakup of his marriage. He says that when he was first married his wife would come to cheer for him and help out at all his bike races, no matter how much travel was involved. But as the marriage became less satisfying and fulfilling for them both, her support diminished, until she would only take him to the airport and pick him up on his return. Because racing bicycles was his occupation, his trips were essential to put bread on the family table, but economy was a reasonable rationale for curtailing her travel.

At first, the routine separations actually seemed to improve the relationship because she developed independent interests. She would meet him at the airline gate with a big hug and a kiss that would congratulate him for winning or console him for losing. If he had fallen in the race he could count on her for sympathy, tender loving care, and help dressing the ugly wounds and road burns. The reunions were romantic, and absence *does* sometimes make the heart grow fonder.

However, the interpersonal conflicts of the marriage were not resolved. The cyclist observed that as the relationship continued to deteriorate, his wife's efforts on behalf of his competition steadily dwindled. She became intolerant of the physical injuries he would occasionally suffer when bikes went down in a race, telling him not to come home if he was all banged up. Gradually his wife would meet him farther and farther away from his plane's arrival gate. Then it was at the curb outside the luggage pickup area. Then it was, "Why don't you grab a cab, honey?" Finally it was, "I don't give a damn how you get home!" Not long after that the marriage ended in divorce.

That's the bad news. On the positive side, many healthy relationships exist in which both partners pursue time-demanding separate activities and also have some interests in common. Endurance sport need not be the dividing wedge, but as one ultradistance cross-country skier put it, it takes a mate "who is extraordinarily understanding to say, 'I understand what you are doing so go to it while you've got enough juice.' " His wife shares many other interests with him, but also directly and indirectly supports his athletics and encourages him to continue enriching his relationships with his training buddies. If endurance sport is a shared interest, then the effect of training will be altogether different from what it is if only one person is an athlete.

And what about parent-child and sibling relationships? What about nonsexual friendships between people of the same or opposite sexes? For that matter, what about friendships between two-legged and four-legged athletes? Far from being the wrecker of homes, endurance sport can provide the cement in the relationship between parent and child, sister and brother, wife and husband. The key is for the people in the relationship to share the activity. No big shock there: people who do things together have that much more opportunity for communication and intimacy.

CHIPS OFF THE OLD BLOCKS

Participation in endurance events by two generations of the same family is not uncommon. What is the effect of a family legacy in ultrasport? Let's take a closer look at three cases: the Erikson, Cates, and Lievanos families.

Did your parents ever bribe you into an accomplishment? Perhaps they promised you a shiny new bicycle if you got all A's, or a baseball glove if you made the team. Jon Erikson remembers that when he was thirteen years old his father, Ted, made him an offer too good to be true: "He asked me if I would like to go to England, and see a little bit of the other countries." Jon immediately responded, "Yeah sure."

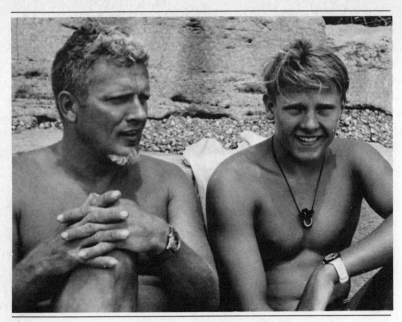

Ted Erikson (left) *and his son, Jon Erikson* (right).

COURTESY OF VERN PETRO

But then his father set the hook: "Well, nothing in this life is for free. I'll be more than glad to finance your trip to England, but you'll have to try to prove yourself, and do something for it." As his father reeled him in, Jon said, "What's that?" Turns out that the only hitch was, when he got to England he would have to swim across the English Channel. The "little bit of the other countries" was the northwestern edge of France.

If your father were anybody but Ted Erikson, striking such a bargain might be tantamount to child abuse. But Ted Erikson was no ordinary father. He had successfully swum a double crossing of the English Channel, and he was serious about helping his son earn the trip to England. The elder Erikson was nearing the end of an illustrious career as a professional endurance swimmer, and perhaps he was ready to pass the baton to his son at a time when their relationship had become more crucial to him than ever before. "I got divorced just about that time. And I was also ready to stop swimming. My son came and lived with me in Chicago, and he was just starting to swim. I had about one or two more years to go. I was just doing the Farallon swim."

The Farallon swim, Erikson's last big swim, was a particularly grueling undertaking. It was a 31-mile slog in the shark-infested, cold Pacific Ocean from tiny Farallon Island to the northern shore of San Francisco's Golden Gate. At least two scuba divers are known to have been attacked by sharks in those waters. (Amazingly, both survived.) Timing is critical since the tide rushing out of the Golden Gate reaches 9 knots at certain hours. During his first attempt to swim from Farallon to the U.S. mainland, the water ranged between 52 and 56 degrees Fahrenheit. After five hours of swimming he passed out from hypothermia and his crew had to pull him aboard the boat. He was lucky to survive. On his second attempt he fell victim to seasickness and succumbed to nausea after ten hours in the water. Finally, on a third try on September 16, 1967, he successfully swam to the Golden Gate Bridge. His time: 14:28.

Ted Erikson was more than just a professional athlete, but it was the athletics that brought him closest to his son. "I was swimming more or less as a diversion from my work, which was too much head stuff. I wanted to get some physical exercise. I was doing government research then, rocket sensitivities, explosive sensitivities, developing new propellants and things like that." Jon, for his part, had been involved in AAU age-group swimming from the time he was ten. However, when the family split-up caused him to move from Ridge Park into Chicago the youngster was also separated from his swim team.

It was natural for swims at the Point—a Lake Michigan park frequented by swimmers—to become a common focus of the Eriksons' life together. "Jon would come out to the lake when I would be finishing a workout, or in a workout," Ted reminisces, "and I'd be kicking on a flutter-board, doing a mile kick. He would swim alongside." In this tadpole phase of Jon's development, he could keep up with his father only because kicking provides less than one-third as much power as does swimming with both arms and legs.

Jon progressed, though, and Ted can still chart his son's improvement: "A little time went by and pretty soon he was getting fast enough so I couldn't kick with him. I would pull with just my arms and he'd be alongside. I made a deal with him that if he wanted to swim the Channel, he'd have to do some rather long lake swimming and prove to me he was serious about it. Pretty soon we could swim even, and then as time went on and I started getting a little older and not doing much swimming anymore, I started wearing fins with him to keep up. There came a time when I couldn't beat him even with fins, so I wound up getting a sailboard and I started sailing alongside of him. He just kept getting better and better and I kept getting worse."

At thirteen, it was time for Jon Erikson to prove his mettle in the English Channel. While his father waited onshore, Jon tried to stroke from England to France. On that first attempt, Jon says, "I didn't have what it takes. I really didn't have enough weight on my body. I just kind of froze up. After about five hours of swimming I was frozen. I couldn't psychologically or physically go on." Another victim of Channel hypothermia.

By endurance-swimming standards, Jon was still a skinny little kid. The totem of the open-water swim clan ought to be the walrus; distance swimmers are much more hefty than their pool-swimming counterparts in the world of sprinting. They typically carry some fat for bouyancy and insulation. Like his father, Jon eventually developed the archetypal endurance swimmer's body. Only five foot ten, at one point he weighed in at 235 pounds.

One year after his first attempt, a somewhat heavier teenager returned to England. This time Ted was unable to accompany his son. After eleven hours and twenty-two minutes, Jon crawled ashore at Cap Gris Nez. Although younger boys have done it since, at that time he was the youngest male to cross the Channel. (An American girl, Lenore Modell, was two months younger than Jon when she swam the Channel in 1964.)

After his very respectable Channel triumph, Jon went on to other glories as a swimmer. The following year his father put him on the international pro circuit. In Canada he swam Lake Saint John (a 24-mile competition) and La Tuque (a 24-hour relay around a one-third-mile loop). He did the La Tuque event three years with different partners. He also competed in Argentina and Mexico on occasion. Ted says, "He got a lot of traveling out of it. Basically covered expenses; you don't get rich on that. It's not a very lucrative profession, but it's kind of fun, and you get a lot of good experience. After he did the Channel, I figured he might as well get some of the payoff, because I felt he was good enough."

Jon *was* good, too. Never good enough to finish on top, but always good enough to be at least in the middle of the pro ranking on the tour, sometimes as high as second. He achieved his major goal, which, according to Ted, was to "do everything that I've done and more."

Ted Erikson had done the double crossing, so after Jon broke his father's double-crossing record by just three minutes, he set his sights on crossing the Channel three times. As Jon puts it, "The triple Channel swim was my last hurrah. I was on the professional circuit for about ten years, and I wasn't doing too bad: making three to five grand a summer sometimes. I loved it. But as the years went by, ex-Olympic swimmers started coming on. They had ex-Olympians from Holland and Yugoslavia and these guys were just speedsters. The handwriting was on the wall. I was doing some of the best times I had ever done in my life at twenty-five years old, and these people were just beating me. So I said, 'Well, either just get out of swimming, or go out with something that is going to make a mark for yourself, and something that's going to be tough for somebody else to beat.' I figured it's got to be cold, it's got to be rough, and it's got to be long. That's why it was the triple Channel, although I was having questions the first two years I tried, '79 and '80, and was unsuccessful. I was really hard-nosed. It was an obsession."

In 1979 Jon was cheated by the Channel's fickle weather. In that region, predicting the weather an hour in advance is sometimes considered a long-range forecast. A triple crossing ought to take at least a day, and in that time the Channel's weather can turn from dead calm to a hurricane. Although conditions were acceptable when he started, toward the end of the third lap the waves were kicking up to about 12 feet. The French call the Channel *La Manche,* because it is in reality "a sleeve" through which flows the tempestuous Atlantic Ocean. The first attempt finally had to be aborted because Jon was slipping backward and the support boat couldn't hold a position near him. During that ill-fated attempt, Jon swam two and three-quarters laps of the Channel.

The next year, 1980, the weather was already turning sour as Jon completed his second lap. A decision was made, on the basis of economics, to forgo a shot at the third lap. Once they enter the water up to their knees, Channel swimmers are financially committed to their boat captains. With the waves kicking up, a repeat of the previous year's experience was very likely. It just didn't make sense to risk wasting the fee of $1,500 per crossing.

Frustration was dogging the project, but inevitably his obsession brought Jon back to Folkestone. In Jon's view, "There's no question: the English Channel has been and probably always will be the proving ground for marathon swimmers, because of all the different things that it can throw at you—the cold water, the currents, the tides, and the weather."

This time when he entered the water at 8:44 A.M. on August 11, 1981, the water was a little choppy, but the 2-foot waves gave way to completely calm seas before the attempt was over. A second difference this time was the presence on board the support boat of Jon's father. Ted Erikson had been absent from all Jon's previous triple-Channel swims, in order to avoid putting any additional pressure on his son. By age twenty-six, however, the thirteen-year veteran of marathon swimming was too experienced for his father's participation to be a distraction.

His first lap, from England to France, took only ten hours and ten minutes. His return from France to England was understandably a bit slower—13:14.

On August 12, 1981, at 11:11 P.M., after thirty-eight hours and twenty-seven minutes of swimming, Jon Erikson became the first person to triple-cross the Channel. At this writing he is the only person to have achieved that feat, which involves over 63 miles of ocean swimming. The final lap, from England to France, had required fifteen hours and three minutes. That lap was Jon's eleventh successful Channel crossing.

So how did all this affect the relationship between father and son? Ted says, "It probably brought us closer together than any two human beings. He wasn't my son, he was my buddy." Jon concurs: "It was an interesting relationship, because he was my dad, but he also was for many, many years, and still is, my best friend."

Ted explains that their present camaraderie was at least partly a consequence of the Eriksons' earlier family situation: "I was divorced, so I wound up getting into trouble—doing a little shenanigans and stuff. Jon watched me do just about everything wrong, and wouldn't say anything, but would always give me support—emotional support." Ted describes a relationship in which father and son swapped roles and both seemed to be better off because of it: "I would count on him for anything. I don't want to bother him with my problems, but he was much more emotionally stable than I was. We used to give these little talks. Because of the swimming we sometimes got in demand on the lecture circuit, and we used to have this little Mutt-and-Jeff act. He was always the straight man; I was the kinky guy. It went across pretty good. Even though he was only fourteen, even that young, he still was much more serious than I was. He was really the father giving stability to the relationship, and I was the wild son."

Then there is the competition to consider, too. Athletic competition between members of a family could conceivably become a divisive factor. That was not the case with the Eriksons, however. According to Jon, "The competition kind of made us grow closer together rather than farther apart. When I broke his record for the two-way he was my sponsor, as far as sending me over there and things like that. It wasn't like anybody was trying to rub anybody's nose in something."

Neither Ted nor Jon now participates in endurance swimming at anything near his previous level. Ted swims a few miles per week for exercise and recreation, but he retired from professional swimming around 1970 and now, at fifty-seven, is an avid sailboarder. Jon retired after the triple crossing in 1981 and briefly took up running, easily reaching a level of 10 miles a day. He competed in one short triathlon recently, finishing in the middle of the pack. At age thirty, Jon's sports interests now include golf and swimming 3 to 4 miles per week.

Though their days of competitive marathon swimming are over, both still pursue athletics to maintain health and fitness. Speaking for them both, Jon says, "Don't get me wrong, I love to sit down and enjoy a football game as much as anybody else, but when it comes to the point that watching a movie or reading a book or doing something like that is a heck of a lot more important than actually getting out there and trying it myself, it's going to be because I don't have any choice."

Perhaps more important than anything else, both Ted and Jon seem to believe that the warmth and strength of their relationship is largely attributable to their mutual pursuit of marathon swimming.

Ken Cates, age fifty-five, does triathlons, along with his sons Michael, thirty-one, and Brian, thirty. Ken is a retired schoolteacher, Michael has a Ph.D. in chemistry and works as a researcher, and Brian is a furniture maker who specializes in finish carpentry for fancy new restaurants. The trio has competed in numerous swim races, bike races, footraces, and triathlons of varying lengths. In 1983 Team Cates, as they sometimes call themselves, competed in the Ironman Triathlon. All three finished.

Endurance sports can make one obsessive. A sports obsession can reach out and grab an athlete for life. You certainly would believe that, if you heard Ken Cates talk of surfing and triathlons: "There are two things that really registered on me in terms of 'athletic pleasure.' One was in 1950. I was walking along the beach with a bunch of guys. We turned a corner and *I saw guys riding long boards.* Something snapped! I said, 'I'm gonna do that. I don't care what it costs me, I'm gonna do that.' The next summer I was working at the beach, and I learned to surf just like that.

"The second thing was that Ty [Hal Tyvoll, an attorney, surfing buddy of Ken's, and triathlete] told me about a little San Diego Track Club short-distance triathlon. That was the mid-seventies and I went out and watched that race. And I thought, 'I'm born to this. I've got to do this.' "

There's a bumper sticker that reads "Insanity is contagious; you catch it from your children." The Cates family's athletic mania is an example of the reverse. Brian explains: "Ken brought us up in the water and on the beach in surfing. He had us out as kids, surfing when we were five years old. I had been surfing probably twenty or twenty-five years, heavily for about fifteen. That's all I did through junior high school, high school, and ten years after. It was the most fun I could ever imagine, but I never competed. To me, surfing is not something you can judge, because they can only judge your style, not who crosses the line first. So I never got to work out my competitiveness. All of a sudden, about five or six years ago, my father and I started to do some 10-k's together. And it became something, to race in a competition."

When Ken discovered the triathlon, he was initially intimidated by the Hawaiian event. The Ironman's 2.4-mile swim, 112-mile bike race, and 26.2-mile footrace seemed like excessive distances. Then a few of his cronies and training buddies did it, and he knew it was possible for properly trained ordinary athletes to finish. So in 1982 he went over to Hawaii and came back with a second-place finish in his division (13:10).

Then the only challenge was how to get his sons to do it with him next year. In order to proselytize for lunacy Ken had to use a campaign of disinformation: "I love to tell stories. So I'd come and b.s. them until their eyes would roll back. With a purpose, though. Maybe I could get them hooked." Pretty soon Ken had Michael and Brian believing that something as painful as the Ironman would actually be fun.

Brian was a pushover, because the competitive-running bug had bitten him, but Michael had dropped athletic activity during his paper chase: "I did surfing for a long time. I got into karate for about five years. And then I sort of quit. I was going to graduate school. I got up to about 205, put on some weight. I didn't do anything for a couple of years. Then I decided to start working out again, and I began to lift weights. I lost some weight, and I felt really good. I felt strong. My neighbor across the street was a woman who was into running. She looked so athletic and nice that I thought, 'God I'd like to get into running.' I started running, and then I didn't think I was that good at it, so I started doing some swims. I prepared for a whole summer to swim Del Mar Days [a 1-mile race in the Pacific Ocean], and I pounded it out pretty good. That was sort of the start, and then I got into doing some 10-k's. At that time Ken was doing triathlons and marathons. I thought there's no way I'd ever run a marathon."

Nonetheless, when Ken came round with his yarns about the Ironman, Michael sounded already ripe for plucking: "For me doing the Ironman was sort of a quest for the ultimate. If you do something, you want to do it first-class, top of the line. Like studying chemistry in school: the top of the line was a Ph.D., so you pound it out and get one of those. For triathlons, it seemed like the Ironman was the pinnacle, and so. . . ." It's not difficult to sell to an achiever if you offer a product as challenging as the Ironman.

A gambler would have predicted that the Cates family team would finish the 1983 Ironman in order of the members' ages, with youngest first. That's not what happened. The youngest, Brian, believes that he went into that race in excellent condition. He had a good swim split (1:23.35), followed by an excellent bike ride (6:10.53). But he didn't drink and eat enough early on, so he had trouble on the run. At mile 3 of the marathon he experienced cold chills. Soon after that stomach cramps and vomiting began. At mile 10 Brian's much slower brother, Michael, trotted past him. The day after the race a local Hawaiian newspaper had two photos on the front page: Dave Scott beating all other Ironmen and Brian Cates looking like a cadaver that had been draped across the hood of a parked car. For Brian, you might say that the Ironman was one of those experiences that builds character. "The hardest part of the race was getting off the car hood and going on with the race." Brian did finish the race after five hours and thirty-eight minutes on the run, but not before his father, twenty-five years his senior, passed him at mile 23.

The Cateses compete with each other in races and when they go out on training rides, and Brian finishes ahead of the rest of the clan more often than not. But as with Ted and Jon Erikson, the competition seems to enhance rather than detract from the relationship. During a recent bicycle event in Mexico, all three were riding in a pack that included some other riders. Drafting—taking turns "pulling" at the front—confers a substantial advantage for the pack over individual riders. The pack attacked a hill. Brian says, "The momentum got going up this hill fairly well. It was a fairly long one, and it was a grinder. We just ground it out and Ken started to fall back. I looked back a couple of times. We got to the top—the flat—and he had lost 50 yards on the hill and started to lose a little more. I looked over at Mike and said, 'It looks like Kenny boy's gonna lose it here.' Mike said, 'Should we drop back and get him?' We looked at each other and said, 'No way.' Mike's comment was, 'Well, you know what he'd do in this situation.' 'That's right,' I said. 'We'll see him in Ensenada.' "

Training and playing together as adults seems to have had a salutary effect on the relationship between father and sons. Ken tries to analyze how their endurance hobby has enhanced the relationship: "I was away from these guys for quite a number of years when I separated from their mom. It was a bad time for everyone involved, and I hoped this might be a pleasant, noncontroversial commonality. It proved to be exactly that; Michael and I are light-years closer. I think I have extricated myself from the role of 'father.' I'm obviously their old man, and I don't let them forget it, but I don't demand a damn thing from them. I don't even want a card on Father's Day. I'm just proud to be their father as well as a buddy."

At present, the three Cateses are waiting for their entry packets for the upcoming Ironman.

Big and Little Alex Lievanos, as they are sometimes called, were split up by the elder Leivanos's divorce. From the time Little Alex was eleven years old, father-and-son contact had largely been confined to holiday and weekend visitations.

At five foot eight, Big Alex weighed in at 175 pounds—not obese, but overweight. His father had died of a heart attack, and eleven years ago one of his friends, a young attorney, also died of a heart attack. Sufficiently scared, Big Alex took up running as a means to reduce his weight and lessen his risk of heart disease. The life-style change stuck; Big Alex became an ultradistance runner. Long-distance runs of as much as 60 miles were not uncommon for Alex. Split workouts totaling more than 20 miles per day became his norm. On February 28, 1981, at age forty-two, Big Alex ran in a 50-mile race at the Grossmont College track in La Mesa, California. (Despite driving rain, Alex won his age division with a time of 7:15.)

There is one part of Big Alex's life-style that didn't change until later. When he first began ultradistance running, he suffered from alcoholism, a disease he has been recovering from since 1981. Remarkably, his alcoholism had not hindered his running; in fact, sometimes he used running as a hangover cure. He also used it to convince himself that he couldn't possibly be an alcoholic. He would tell himself, "Alcoholics can't run 75 miles," and then he would go on with his drinking binge.

Not long after he completed the drying-out phase of his recovery at a hospital, Big Alex took a vacation in Hawaii to watch his friend Ken Cates compete in the Ironman. As so often happens, watching the event infected him with a case of triathlon fever.

By this time Big Alex was occasionally running with his seventeen-year-old son. "Little Alex had been living with my first wife and had been experiencing emotional and behavioral difficulties with his mother. She was getting ready to throw him out on the street. So he came to live with Diane and me at the beach."

When Big Alex got a crazy gleam in his eye and suggested that the two of them train for the Ironman, his son agreed readily. Of course there were some problems to overcome. The father had very little cycling experience. That didn't deter him though: "I went and bought two bicycles and all the equipment that went with them. I had never been on a ten-speed bike in my life, but I decided to ride the bike from the shop to my place. My first real bike ride, and I fell over. I hadn't thought about the bike being such a tricky machine, and having to recondition all my old joints and muscles. By the time we got through training to go to Hawaii, my son and I were riding from Pacific Beach to San Clemente and back every Saturday. That's a hundred-mile round trip."

Then there was the challenge of swimming. Big Alex had a graceful style, but lacked the requisite swimming endurance to navigate 2.4 miles. On the other hand, Little Alex had a very choppy sprinter's style, but he had the strength and endurance to thrash his way through. Somehow they both improved.

But there is a sad twist to this story. At first Big Alex tried to deny to himself that illness was creeping up on him. When the headaches and vague pains turned into vomiting the day before the race, it was no longer possible to attribute the malaise to Hawaii's humid, energy-draining climate. After the emergency-room doctor completed his tests, the indictment came back: "You have a virus. You have a fever of 102 and you're dehydrated." The rejoinder: "Give me a shot or something and fix me up so I can do this thing tomorrow." This physician had been around Kona a long time, and this probably was not the first ironman he'd ministered to. The verdict: "You're sick. You've got a fever. You just can't."

Despite all resolve to the contrary, on race day Big Alex couldn't get out of bed. He shook hands with Little Alex and sent him off with, "I can't do this, so good luck." Big Alex was able to make it to the race course, although he was not well enough to stay for the finish. "Just to know he was there watching me made me feel good." Little Alex finished with a time of 13:48.

Did endurance training have an emotional effect? Little Alex says, "It took a lot of togetherness to do something like that. My father inspired me." The father's words also describe what training together did for the relationship: "The normal paternal love that one would expect between a father and son was greatly enhanced by training for that endurance event, because of the shared experience, suffering through the pain together. We wore out the tires together, we wore out our spirits together, we wore out our bodies together, we rebuilt them together, we ate together, we nurtured each other, we supported each other emotionally, spiritually.

"Because of my alcoholism, I feel we did not have the kind of father-son relationship I would have liked to have had. I accept responsibility for that, because I am an alcoholic. I've tried to make up for the lack of a solid relationship. I'm sure there's an element of overcoming guilt, but the important thing is that I've made the effort.

"Because of the training we went through, I later was able to share with my son very honestly. Because of the experience, I can speak man-to-man to my son now. It's opened up the communication channel. I've been able to advise my son on important decisions. He wouldn't have sought my advice without that experience."

Athletic training enhances awareness of physical feelings, even if only the feelings of pain and fatigue. People who train together are experiencing the same level of pain, elation, fatigue, so they learn to empathize in the most direct and elementary manner possible. Hence, the workouts give training buddies the opportunity to practice communicating their feelings with each other. That's expressing a *feeling*, albeit a physical feeling. It's not such a great step to shift to the emotional feelings, and the ability to communicate innermost emotions is considered the cornerstone of intimacy.

Big Alex also thinks there's "some kind of chemistry that happens" between blood relatives. He is intrigued by the spiritual connection between siblings, fathers and sons, and other kin: "What kind of a nurturing relationship existed at the time? Can it be identified? Was it support, was it coercion, was it ass kicking, was it embarrassment or humiliation, was it competition? 'You think you can beat your old man; watch this!' "

The benefits of training together were tangible as well as emotional, according to Big Alex: "I felt my son did not have a very good image of himself. I wanted to enhance him as a person through this physical activity; not only physical activity, but an elite physical activity. The Ironman championships in Hawaii! This is the ultimate! So we took on the big one, and we made it. When Little Alex came back from Hawaii he went out and got a job just like that. He was feeling like a champ and he was. He felt very potent, very powerful.

"Considering the relationship from the time of Alex's birth until the present, our Ironman training has got to be the high point. There are events like certain Christmases, or his first bike, or the first time he caught a fish—but in terms of a major decision and commitment to do something together, this has got to be it. I'm really proud that I was able to do that with him."

AM I MY BROTHER'S TRAINER?

Jeff and Scott Tinley are brothers who often have trained and competed together in triathlons. Scott, the elder of the two by three years, won the Ironman Triathlon in both 1982 and 1985. In the 1982 race, Jeff came in third. In other shorter triathlons the Tinley brothers have taken the first two positions.

Sylviane and Patricia Puntous are identical twins. If you see them out training in their matching outfits, you could easily believe that you are seeing double. The two French Canadians have dominated women's triathlon competition for the past several years. The Puntous twins are accustomed to finishing one, two, not infrequently holding hands, because they are in a dead heat for the victory.

At the 1983 Ironman some miscreant sabotaged the bicycle course with carpet tacks, and Patricia Puntous fell victim to flat-tire problems.

Her sister regretted leaving her behind, but it was that or risk both of them losing the race. Sylviane went on to win that Ironman with a time of 10:43.39. Patricia fixed her tire and still managed to come in second, only six minutes behind her sister (the time it took her to fix her flat). The twins had to run the entire 26.2-mile footrace without any contact or chance to pace each other. Remarkably, when final results were reported, it was learned that their marathon times differed by only five seconds. Uncanny!

Clearly something extraordinary happens when siblings participate jointly in endurance sports.

When Larry Krieger talked his sister Lois into being his handler for the Ricoh East Coast Triathlon Championship in October 1983, he probably had no idea what he was starting. Lois, now thirty-three, is a book editor who, at the time, did some swimming and running, but didn't even own a bike. Larry, now twenty-seven, had just started medical school.

There is something about endurance athletics that seems to impel spectators to become participants. Perhaps it is because most of the spectators know one or more of the contestants, so it's impossible to avoid empathizing. The typical endurance event is not at all like a football or basketball game, something being done by highly paid gladiators—a class of humans apart from ourselves. Endurance athletics is something done by ordinary, flesh-and-blood friends, neighbors, lovers, or relatives—folk we know personally. It's easy to feel remote from the stars of spectator sports, but it's impossible to view a triathlon or marathon and not imagine yourself going through the same motions as the loved one you came to cheer and support. Lois felt bad about watching rather than doing, so Larry was easily able to convince her to train for the following season.

Lois and Larry come from a relatively unified family, but the two of them had not been particularly close at the time they embarked on their triathlon training. Lois is six years older than Larry, so she had felt the normal maternal feelings older sisters typically feel for their younger brothers. However, as Lois tells it, "I went away to school while he was a teenager and missed his formative years. When I came back for visits, I didn't see him much. When I did, I didn't particularly like him. He was a rotten teenager, a lot wilder than I was. I didn't understand him and didn't spend much time with him."

Maturation does wonderful things. As Larry entered his twenties and Lois passed into her late twenties, the age gap narrowed and they drew closer to each other. Says Larry, "We could share things on an equal level for the first time."

The brother and sister trained together during the next year. They

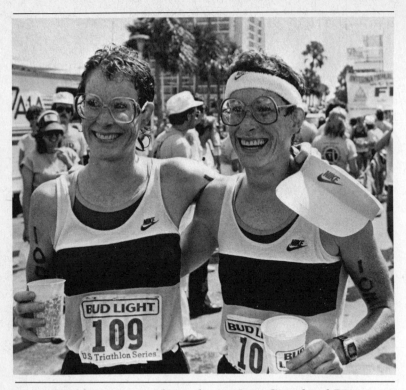

Double exposure. Identical twins Jann Girard and Dian Girard-Rives finished one-two at the 1985 Fort Lauderdale USTS race. COURTESY OF BUD LIGHT USTS

set as their season-end goal the 1984 Cape Cod Endurance Triathlon, an Ironman-length event. Training was the perfect activity for the summer between Larry's first and second year of medical school. Lois bought a bike and they rode and ran together whenever they could on the roads near their parents' house in New Jersey. There is a lake nearby, where they did their swimming. They entered eight shorter triathlons that summer. As their training progressed in July and August of 1984, their relationship changed too. Lois says, "I suddenly didn't want to spend as much time in New York, or with my friends, because I wanted to rush back home—partially to train and partially to be with Larry, because we had become so close. I was seeing someone at the time, and yet it took back seat to what we were doing. I tried to work my social schedule around the training Larry and I had planned for the weekend. My friend didn't mind because he knew how important it was to me."

The Kriegers prepared adequately for the 1984 Cape Cod Triathlon. They swam and put in the long miles on the bike and road that summer, training as much as six or seven hours per day. They did a

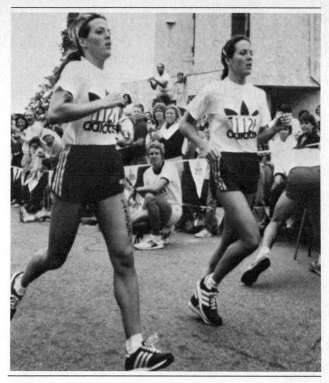

Sylviane and Patricia Puntous finishing in a dead heat for first at the Los Angeles USTS Triathlon.

shorter triathlon nearly every other weekend. Just one week prior to the event Larry suffered some injuries when an automobile ran his bicycle off the road. Nonetheless, they both competed and Larry was even able to play on the crowd's sympathy by wearing bandages on the two fingers he broke in the bike accident.

These ultradistance events have a life-long emotional impact on many participants, particularly when they are done with friends and loved ones. Take Lois Krieger's reaction, for example: "This is very corny, but one of the nicest feelings I ever had was when I crossed the finish line at Cape Cod. There was a lot going on there: TV cameras, lights, music. But the greatest thing when I crossed the line was that Larry was already there, and he hugged me and said, 'I can't believe it, we actually did it.' There was this big look of accomplishment and pride on his face, and I felt the pride was for my accomplishment as well as his. It was such a good feeling because it was something we did together, something we achieved that we never before thought we could achieve."

Larry's innocent suggestion at the Ricoh event has created a monster. Lois plans to continue competing in triathlons. "I'm hoping we're going to keep doing these kinds of things for a long time, until we get into the older age groups and can start winning some awards."

Triathlon training has made a substantial difference in the sibling relationship. Larry now consults Lois "about things [he] would normally only talk to friends about." Lois has noticed they telephone each other frequently. "I don't remember us ever calling each other just to chat in the past, whereas we've done that this year." On weekends when both Kriegers are at the family home, they work alongside each other—Lois on freelance editing, Larry on his medical studies—and then they take breaks to train or consume large quantities of food.

Of course Larry and Lois, or anybody else who trains with a family member, spouse, or lover, could spend the same amount of time doing some other activity together, something intellectual perhaps. But the Kriegers agree that the result would not have been nearly so favorable to the relationship as the triathlon training has been. Lois explains: "It was something so purely physical. Writing or studying doesn't quite give you the same feeling of achievement as physical accomplishment. There's more pressure with intellectual pursuits, whereas, if it's purely physical, it's sharing good times."

Very likely the Kriegers will continue to "share the good times" in triathlons. For Lois "it's a matter of having discovered something I love to do, and want to continue to do forever." The relationship between Larry and Lois has been profoundly altered by training together for endurance sport. Nonetheless, the bottom line is that they got closer together because what they did together was just plain fun.

TWO CAN TRAIN AS CHEAPLY AS ONE

It was bound to happen sooner or later, and finally in 1985 it did. Ken and Lisa Martin from Mesa, Arizona, entered the Pittsburgh Marathon together. Ken won the men's race with a time of 2:12.57. Lisa took the women's competition with a time of 2:31.52. This is probably the first time that a husband-and-wife team made a clean sweep of a major marathon.

Of course it is not so strange for couples to pursue endurance sport together. But what's the effect of that? The Norwegian runner Grete Waitz and her coach/husband Jack Waitz come to mind immediately as one couple for whom joint participation in athletics seems to have led to a closer relationship. (Grete, who has won five world cross-country championships and once held the women's world record in the marathon, also trains with her brother Jan, who used to be one of the best cross-country skiers in Norway.) On the other hand, runners

Mary Decker and Ron Tabb received nearly as much publicity for their divorce as they have for running. In general, though, common sense suggests that couples enhance their relationships when they share an activity as challenging as endurance athletics.

Tamalpais is a rugged little mountain in Marin County, California, on the peninsula that anchors the northern end of the Golden Gate Bridge. Although Tamalpais is a midget among the world's mountains, it is a steep little devil; it very precipitously rises to 2,600 feet from a base at near sea level. The infamous 13.6-mile Double Dipsea Footrace, with its 5,200 feet of vertical climb, takes place on the trails that crisscross the slopes of Mount Tamalpais. For a number of years now, a group of forty or fifty long-distance runners has congregated at Mount Tamalpais on Saturday mornings in order to do hillwork.

Mary Ann Buxton, a forty-three-year-old athletics-clothing consultant and manufacturer, believes that the Tamalpais group is social and recreational as well as serious about running. Mary observes, "There always is a lot of dating that goes on out of that group. A lot of relationships have developed, some that have been maintained, some that have not, and some that have switched." Mary Ann ought to know: she and the man she loves, Tom Barthold, met on one of these Mount Tamalpais runs.

Tom Barthold, a management consultant, whose friends call him Bart, is now forty-two years old. At the time Bart met Mary Ann, he had recently done the Western States 100-Miler. His description of their courtship sounds like a cross between *Love Story* and a training diary: "When I stood up there on the starting line I had absolutely no doubt in my mind that I was going to finish the race. Right in the middle I start thinking, 'What can I do next? This race is over, I've only got another twelve hours or so to go.' I had read the article in *Sports Illustrated* about the Ironman. I said, 'Why not? I'm a good runner, I'm a good swimmer, and all I have to do is learn to bicycle.' So I was already planning my training for the Ironman, while I was running the Western States.

"Not long after that I met Mary Ann. All she had done was a few marathons and was really not very focused in her training.

"I was thirty-seven then, and I'd never been married. I couldn't find anybody I enjoyed being with that much, who was interested in sports and good health. All the female athletes I was around were already taken. I didn't like the idea of hanging out in bars, so finally I just stopped worrying about it. I said, 'It will just happen, doing what I'm doing now.' And practically the next week she was there running. She had been with us before up on Mount Tam on Saturday morning runs, and I guess when you just least expect it you notice things.

"We were talking about training, and I said that I was training for a triathlon, and she said, 'Oh, I've done a triathlon.' I was surprised to find anybody had done triathlons. Later I did the one she had done and I won it. She said, 'Well, what are you going to do now?' I said, 'I think I'll go to Davis and do the triathlon.' She said, 'Well, I'll go to Davis and do it too.' I said, 'But that's a mile swim.' She said, 'I can do a mile swim.' She could do the breaststroke, and that was it. I was surprised at her lack of concern.

"We did Davis, and I did real well up there. Then she said, 'Now what?' And I said, 'The only other triathlon that's around is Hawaii.' She said, 'Yeah, I think I'll go to Hawaii.' I said, 'That's 2.4 miles; how are you gonna swim that?' She said, 'I guess I'll have to learn how to swim.' She had been telling me about the ride and ties. She said, 'I'll make a deal with you: I'll learn to swim if you learn to ride a horse.' "

Bart and Mary kept their bargain. Bart learned to ride, and so far the couple has teamed up on three Levi's Ride and Ties. Mary says that Bart has "probably kept his part of the deal better than I have. He's gone on to be a better rider and even more enthusiastic about the horses than I am, whereas I'm still a plodder on the cycling and the swimming." Mary may be too modest: she has competed quite well in the five Ironman Triathlons that she has done with Bart. And, oh, yes, they got married in 1981. The ceremony took place at Rock Springs Meadow, one of the couple's favorite places on Mount Tamalpais.

Bart had found a partner who shared his passion for endurance sport. As he sees it, "She had the same attitude that I had. I guess I really didn't expect it in a woman—never verbalizing any limitations: 'Got a new event; sure, let's go do it.' "

For her part, Mary was also glad to find somebody like Bart. So many of her previous boyfriends had been unsupportive of her interest in sports. "It seemed to be something they were in competition with." They resented the time commitment, and Mary's ability may have threatened the machismo of some of her previous beaux. "Looking back, before I started to compete in running and triathlons, every fall I would lose a boyfriend because ski season would start." Mary's pattern was to meet somebody in the spring or summer who would tell her how much he loved skiing and what a wonderful skier he was. Then, as she recalls, "Ski season would come around and we'd go skiing, and he couldn't stand that I could fly down the slopes, that I was an excellent skier. It would always interfere with the relationship.

I never had any patience with men who couldn't handle my competence in whatever I did."

Nothing's perfect, and it would be foolish to assume that Bart and Mary never have the sorts of disagreements that inevitably plague all couples. Even though they train together and go to the same races, they have decided to attack the actual competition separately. For one thing, their pace is different. (Bart's best marathon time is 2:48 and Mary's is about 3:25.) For another, they have learned that they sometimes endure pain better separately.

Bart, who was a more experienced ultradistance runner than Mary, tried to pace her through her first ultramarathon, the American River 50-Miler. "It was a complete disaster," Bart recalls, "and that's why I won't run with her anymore." He believes "it's very helpful the first time you run an ultra to have someone pace you. It's so time-consuming, and you need to control your speed carefully at the beginning of the race. You feel so good and so fit, you don't like to be going at that slow a speed. So I thought I would help her out. I wanted to run well there, but, feeling unselfish, I thought, 'I'll pace her through this.' "

The road to hell is paved with good intentions. Bart meant well, but the experience he describes just didn't turn out that way: "As we got going and she started falling apart, she would say things like, 'Why did you ever let me run this?' She became critical of everything I was saying. I'd say, 'No, you're doing fine, let's walk a little bit.' She'd say, 'I'm not doing fine.' I was taking these remarks pretty personally. Fine, I thought, anything I say is disastrous, so I won't say anything. That's not what you have somebody along talking to you for, so I couldn't be that functional anymore.

"Everything I did was wrong. It was so frustrating. A guy came up and he said, 'You think we're gonna make it in under ten hours?' I looked at my watch and I said, 'No, I don't think so.' After the guy left Mary Ann said, 'Well, that's a hell of a thing to say to somebody, he can't make it under ten hours.' I said, 'If I told the guy that he could make it under ten hours, and he took off at a fast pace, he wouldn't even finish the race. At least now I'm sure he's gonna finish.' She said, 'You didn't give him any encouragement.' I said, 'Screw it, I don't even want to talk to you anymore.' And she said, 'Why don't you go off and run by yourself!'

"She was crying and really feeling sorry for herself. So I went off and just kind of sprinted for the next 10 miles or so. I felt wonderful; then I started feeling guilty that I left her out there. So I sat under a tree and waited for her to come along. We finished together.

"I think she was feeling better that I wasn't there. She takes her adversity better when I'm not around. That was also pretty early in our relationship. And she had a lot of physical problems, a lot of cramping. She felt a lot better the next day. We were speaking again— I forget pretty rapidly, and so does she—but I made a vow never to pace her again. And I think that works better. The pacer feels obligated, the pacee feels obligated, and it's a difficult situation all around."

Bart and Mary Ann learned that it is preferable to compete independently, but they do train together. Mary explains how: "Bart is a much better athlete than I am. He runs faster, he cycles faster, he swims faster. But he's also a social creature. There's a way we always stay together if we're out cycling. If he's feeling hot, he just takes off. We plan the route so we can reunite, stop for some water, and then take off again. I love to see how I'm improving by how close I am to his time."

Keeping the same pace poses less difficulty on training runs. Both Mary and Bart appreciate the opportunity to communicate. "We use our runs to talk about things," says Bart. His theory is that "there's a tremendous amount of openness early on between runners. We just seem to talk better while we're training."

Mary and Bart enjoy traveling to competitions. Mary explains the routine: "We usually go to the same events. We have what we call the sportsmobile, a van outfitted like a camper. We take the dogs, the bikes, and whatever equipment we're going to use, and take off. We camp out the night before the event and then participate."

They have no present plans to have children. "If Bart and I had met ten years earlier there would be no question," Mary says, "but right now it's not my focus. Maybe in another ten years we'll adopt some kids."

Their present athletic focus is the Western States 100-Miler. Mary was chosen by the lottery—participation is limited to lessen environmental impact—but Bart lost out. He'll go this year as Mary's support crew. This will be her first 100-miler. After that, who knows? Perhaps the Paris-Brest-Paris bike race. Bart has some thoughts about trying a 200-mile wilderness run in Alaska. It's totally unsupported. You have to carry everything, and up there you might need just about anything. One thing seems certain though—they will continue to be endurance athletes. It has become their way of life.

THE LIMITS OF ENDURANCE

PART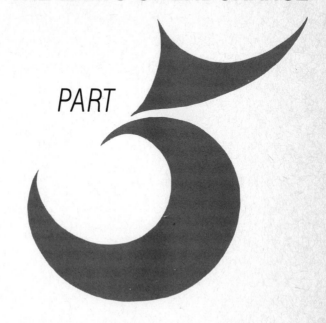

LIMITS

THE MOST exciting and fascinating phenomena in any endurance contest occur inside the minds and bodies of the athletes. The cardiovascular and pulmonary systems, the muscular and skeletal systems, and the subcellular fuel-synthesizing and fuel-burning mechanisms all work together efficiently. It's no wonder Isaac Asimov called his science fiction novel about a journey within the human body *The Fantastic Voyage*. The beautiful harmony with which the body's systems work could lead to the conclusion that anything is possible for an athlete, given balanced, intelligent training, optimum nutrition, the right attitude, and perfect environmental conditions. Is there, in fact, no limit to human endurance?

The human body is so adaptable to hard work that it would be tempting to say that human endurance is limitless. Yet the limits of endurance *do* exist, although they are very difficult to define clearly and precisely. While athletes continue to push back the limits by completing increasingly grueling events in ever faster times, the negative effects of taking the human body to its natural limits are starting to be seen. What then are the physiological and psychological limitations of endurance performance?

The mental and physical aspects are difficult to separate. Hours, months, and sometimes years of dedication are required to excel at endurance sport. Training is long, arduous, time-consuming, and often just plain painful. The pain and dedication that are involved in such training place the limits in the gray area between what is physiological and what is psychological. The tolerance of pain is not something that is easily explained in physiological terms, and the drive to excel in endurance sport is a psychological aspect that inexplicably affects the physiological. It will be decades before exercise scientists and psychologists begin to understand how the psychology of the endurance athlete affects the physiology of the athlete. There is much speculation among scientists about the existence of brain biochemicals that enhance athletic performance. Until these things are better understood, any discussions of physiological and psychological limits are bound to overlap.

PHYSIOLOGICAL BOUNDARIES

The physiological limits in endurance athletics are difficult to identify, except in extreme terms. If a limit is an end, a boundary, an absolute stopping point, and we could list an end point for each type of athletic contest, this topic could be treated very briefly. Exerting oneself to the point of death is an extreme limit, and not very useful to discuss. It is somewhere between dropping dead and sitting around and never attempting any activity that we will find our limits. Since human beings and human bodies are involved in these sports, the definition will be nebulous and must be set on a continuum.

It is possible to discuss a limit in terms of the endurance event itself, e.g., that a two-hour marathon is conceivable, but a one-hour marathon is not. There is no necessary physiological barrier that should make running a sub-two-hour marathon impossible, but the fact that new marathon records are set so infrequently suggests that world-class marathoners may already be taxing their bodies to near the limit of endurance. On the other hand, elite athletes run those races about twice as fast as most human beings can ever run, and still that speed is only about half as fast as a 100-meter sprinter can go.

More than one prediction about the ultimate limits of human performance has proved far too modest. In 1966 B. B. Lloyd wrote in *Advancement of Science* that George Littlewood's 623-mile total for the six-day footrace would probably never be broken. Since the record had stood since 1888, this might have seemed reasonable. After all, until the late 1970s no modern promoter was even conducting any six-day races. Once six-day competition resumed, however, it only took until 1984 for Yiannis Kouros to set the new record, 635 miles. Doubtless, some people may regard the new mark as an absolute upper limit for that event, but Yiannis Kouros is not among those pessimists. He believes that eventually somebody will run as much as 1,200 kilometers (744 miles) in six days. In the case of endurance sport, one always should be reluctant to say that the top has been reached.

Limiting Factors

When talking about limits, it is more useful to talk about the various factors that constrain performance than it is to discuss what is impossible. Boundaries are imposed by the human body and environmental conditions. The many factors that limit an athlete's performance include an inherited biomechanical and aerobic predisposition to excel despite physical hardship; the process of hydration and dehydration; the need for optimum body fueling (proper nutrition); the mysterious need for sleep; and the health effects of training and participating in endurance events.

Inheritance.   Unfortunately, for those of us who fantasize about being a Grete Waitz or Carlos Lopes, an inherited predisposition for outstanding athletic performance may be a major boundary. The limitation imposed by genetics has always been perceived most easily in sprint races and other track-and-field events, such as the high jump and the shotput. It has been popularly believed that training might account for the lion's share of the performance differences in long-distance competition. Recent studies, however, show that aerobic capacity may be largely an inherited quality.

Aerobic capacity is influenced much more by genetics than by gender or age, which is in some sense encouraging. That means we are far less likely to be limited by age than by the genetic material that resides in the cells of our bodies. Not that such late bloomers as Sister Marion Irvine, the nun who qualified for the 1984 Olympic marathon trials at the age of fifty-four, should be any less inspiring, but the potential may have been in their genes all along. Those of us born with the biomechanical advantage (built for speed) and those of us born with a high aerobic capacity (built for endurance) may become the record setters.

Generally speaking, the athletes who exhibit the best performances in endurance sports are small people. There seems to be a body-type specificity for world-class marathon runners just as there is for superb basketball and football players. It isn't too likely that we will see the center for the Sixers running a two-and-a-half-hour marathon. Marathon runners, triathletes, and the like tend to be very spare, lean individuals who aren't very tall. Certainly, the rigor of endurance sport training partly accounts for their spareness, but not all people who train for a marathon become as lean as those we see finishing in the lead pack.

The muscles of elite endurance runners also seem programmed genetically to do exactly what they do—run very far and relatively fast. Just as aerobic capacity might be largely genetically predetermined, so too may be the vascularization that will be possible in an individual's muscles. Vascularization is the extent to which collateral capillaries have been developed to carry blood from arteries to the individual muscle cells. The more capillaries you have, the more efficiently will the oxygen and nutrients reach the muscle cells to produce energy and motion. Training is thought to increase the extent of collateral circulation, but again genetics seems to predetermine how much your body will respond to training by producing the additional blood channels.

A second inherited characteristic of muscles may also determine endurance performance. There are two types of muscle fiber: slow-twitch and fast-twitch. We all have some fibers of each type in our muscles, but the proportion of fast- and slow-twitch fibers varies with each individual. Muscle biopsies of successful sprinters and long-distance athletes have generally shown that sprinters have a higher proportion of fast-twitch fibers and long-distance athletes have a higher proportion of slow-twitch fibers. Fast-twitch fibers, which have a white appearance similar to the white meat of a turkey, metabolize fuel already stored in the fiber, and thus can burn only for quick, anaerobic bursts. (Anaerobic means without air.) Slow-twitch fibers are brown, like the dark meat of a turkey, and can work for extended periods because they obtain their fuel from glycogen and fatty acids in the blood. Depending on what proportion you have of the two types of muscle fiber, you may have more potential as either a sprinter or an endurance athlete.

In sum, every body system has its own genetic program, and that may cause an individual to develop in a manner favorable or unfavorable to endurance performance. World-class endurance athletes may be born with programs that are optimal for the types of athletes they become. Of course, they still have to train, and when two athletes have equal potential the one who works harder probably will be the one who wins.

Some well-known world-class athletes were groomed from very early ages to participate in their sports. Why? Often their parents had been very good at the sport, and they were urged to get involved. Besides receiving encouragement, people who have an athletic legacy may do well because of their inherited body systems. Undeniably, early participation favors development of any inherited predisposition, but here again the heritage is an extra advantage. People whose parents practice a sport are likely to follow the example set by their folks.

Within the genetic limits there isn't much that can keep *anyone* from becoming an endurance athlete, short of pulmonary or heart disease. With proper training, most healthy humans can complete their cross-country ski race or marathon, and anyone can increase his or her speed, working for that personal best. Sports publications are filled with training techniques, and experienced endurance athletes are generally quite eager to help interested novices. Natural selection, however, is what takes world-class athletes into that world class and keeps the rest of us fantasizing about hitting the tape first.

Heat Dissipation and Dehydration.   No matter what your genetic makeup, everyone suffers if the external environment conditions are less than optimum. One crucial factor that affects every athlete's performance is the ability to dissipate heat. The body has three heat-

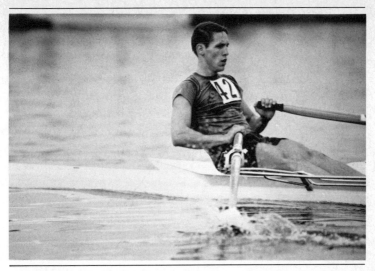

Though clearly working up a sweat, this fit sculler apparently is well within his limits.   PHOTO BY BUDD SYMES

dissipating mechanisms: radiation, evaporation, and conduction. Because internal body temperature can rise so quickly, the optimum external temperature for a record-setting performance in any endurance sport is quite low—in the mid-forties. George Sheehan, a physician who runs and writes about his sport, has said only partly facetiously that if you go out the door to run your marathon and you start sweating before you've run a step, you should turn around and forget the marathon. The critical factor on hot days is dehydration. It will bring the best-trained athlete to a painful stop. Runners or cyclists can sweat away about 4 percent of their body weight within two hours. Rehydration is essential.

It is fairly common to experience moderate to severe muscle cramps after about 20 miles of a marathon. Dehydration is the primary cause. Muscle cells simply lack sufficient water to carry on their vital business under this kind of stress. Thirst usually lags behind the body's need for fluid, so endurance athletes must be careful to rehydrate even before they feel their body signals. It's a good idea for endurance athletes to start drinking lots of water a day or so prior to a race or long workout. A cup of water about fifteen minutes before the start of a race and water taken at intervals of about every 2 miles can help maintain close to a reasonable level of hydration. No athlete will *ever* finish a race completely hydrated, so there is little danger of consuming too much water during a long race.

Nutrition.   There is much discussion these days about the right sort of diet for maximizing endurance and athletic performance. Unlike genetics, nutrition is something that can be controlled by athletes. Diet is now considered by many to be an integral part of the training regimen. The terms "carbohydrate loading" and "glycogen stores" are uttered even by relative novices. Nutrition books such as Robert Haas's *Eat to Win* and Covert Bailey's *Fit or Fat* have become best-sellers.

About a decade ago an interviewer asked marathoner Bill Rodgers what he eats, and Rodgers responded that he could eat anything he wanted. (Apparently he does, too; he reputedly puts mayonnaise on his pizza.) Shortly after Julie Leach won the women's division of the 1982 Ironman Triathlon, a member of the audience at a panel discussion asked her what sort of diet she follows. Julie replied, "I'm on a seefood diet; anything I see, I eat." Despite these answers, it is widely believed that nutrition profoundly influences athletic performance.

Diets high in complex carbohydrates—fruits, vegetables, whole grains—and relatively low in protein and fat are now the order of the day. To maximize endurance performance you don't have to become a vegetarian, but today's conventional wisdom is that it helps to lean in that direction. High-carbohydrate diets maximize the storage of muscle glycogen, that crucial and all-too-easily depleted fuel. Endurance athletes on rigorous training schedules may be able to get by eating anything they want, but they are more likely to eat foods that make them feel fresh and light. Four-time Ironman winner Dave Scott limits his fat intake to low-fat cottage cheese, which he washes before eating in order to remove still more of the fat. Scott's measures may be extreme, but clearly diets high in complex carbohydrates help athletes endure the stress of their sports for the longest possible time.

For endurance events that require refueling during the race, steaks will never do. While competing, athletes typically eat food that can be very quickly metabolized—and that means such items as cookies, candy, and fruit. The sugar in those foods is rapidly transformed to glycogen. The body can burn other fuels besides glycogen, such as fat and even muscle tissue itself. But muscles work best when they can use a combination of fuels; they don't like to work exclusively on fats, and the burning of muscle tissue itself is autocannibalism, a very poor alternative. The medical term for autocannibalism is "tissue necrosis," which means death of the tissue. The risk of tissue necrosis is one reason to avoid total depletion of glycogen stores at all costs. Tissue necrosis obviously does not enhance physical fitness, so it is wise to judiciously schedule participation in endurance events to permit replenishment. If you go into the race nutritionally depleted, your muscles have to get their fuel somewhere.

Sleep.   Some endurance events disrupt normal sleep cycles because they require more than twenty-four hours or even several days. During events such as the bicycle Race Across AMerica and six-day footraces, athletes report hallucinations and other serious manifestations of sleep deprivation (although they seem to recover far more easily than from tissue necrosis). It would be nice to be able to explain why performance deteriorates after long periods without sleep, but no one knows. As yet, sleep researchers do not even know why human beings need to sleep at all. It is known that regular periods of sleep are vital to normal brain function, but what causes sleep onset and what sleep does for us are only partly understood. Depression may possibly be associated with loss of sleep.

Training.   Notions about training, and the optimal training for record-breaking performances, have changed dramatically in recent years. Although the achicvements of world-class athletes convince us that the human body is capable of astounding things, some experts recommend doing no more than two events comparable to a marathon each year. George Sheehan advocates limiting marathon participation to once a year. Frank Shorter has said that a marathoner needs to wait until he or she has forgotten how badly the last marathon hurt. On the other hand, large cash prizes goaded some of the famous nineteenth-century pedestrians to compete in twenty or more ultra-marathons per year, and they were able to maintain that level of participation for decades. In 1984, Yiannis Kouros competed in numerous ultramarathons and two world-record six-day races.

Nevertheless, trainers, coaches, orthopedic surgeons, and other athletic specialists now advocate much shorter training distances and far less intense training workouts than previously, in order to reduce injuries and illness for the endurance athlete. It is difficult to prescribe training limits because they vary according to the individual and are not discrete and clear. There will always be people who can train more intensely than others. But overtraining has prevented some potentially great athletes from achieving the success for which they seemed destined. Endurance athletes seem to do best by alternating hard workouts with easy workouts. If an athlete puts in more than three hard workouts per week, the chances increase that he or she will be injured. Combining speedwork, strength training, and distance work is the optimum way to achieve the record-breaking performance or the personal best time.

Overtraining is an area where psychological limitation may be even more of a problem than physiological. Endurance athletes are often driven, compulsive people who are naturally very competitive. If an athlete hears of a competitor who is putting in more mileage, or more training of any kind, it may be difficult to hold back and avoid working out too hard or too long. The athlete can be trapped in a classic double bind: improvement seems to require more training, but extra training leads to injuries, which prevent training at all. Even if the athlete understands that overtraining is counterproductive, he or she may be unable to accurately discriminate between hard and easy workouts. That is one of the reasons world-class endurance athletes have coaches and trainers to help them plan an optimum individual training program. Some endurance experts believe that Joan Benoit won the women's Olympic marathon in 1984 because a knee injury forced her to rest more and do less rigorous workouts in the weeks prior to the event.

Other similar tales about training convey the same message—less may in fact be more. Triathlete and ultramarathoner Tom Barthold used to run in excess of 70 miles per week. More recently he experimented with running a marathon on only 26 miles per week. He made sure that his workouts included "quality miles" and speedwork. The result was a 2:48 marathon, a personal record for him. Admittedly, his previous running and long background in competition gave him training to fall back on, but the lesson from Barthold's experience seems to be: train smarter not harder.

Maximizing Performance

When Matthew Webb swam the English Channel in a time of 21:45, the world lauded him for achieving the impossible. Yet in a little more than a century the time required for that swim decreased by 65 percent. A similar story can be told about virtually every endurance-sport record. But improvements in the records now come in smaller and smaller increments.

Nonetheless, the physiological boundaries of endurance *are* still being pushed back. Only now the sheer grit of the individual endurance athlete is less responsible than previously for the improvement. Society as a whole has taken an interest in endurance and deserves a small portion of the credit. Although the mind-boggling feats of individual athletes are still essential to improve performance, athletes are not working alone. The scientific community, coaches, trainers, doctors, and other athletes are all looking for ways to maximize endurance performance and minimize the risk of injury or illness. The recently publicized practice of blood doping, the "natural" but controversial way to introduce more oxygen-carrying hemoglobin into the blood of world-class athletes, is very likely only a preview of the kinds of alterations we may see in the regimens of athletes. Just as our society has become more technologically sophisticated in the nonathletic sphere, computers are being introduced to help design training programs for athletes. Certainly those most interested in top performance will continue to search for new, natural, and legal ways to break through the physiological limits.

PSYCHOLOGICAL BOUNDARIES

One cyclist performs better in competition than in training. A rowing crew seems to experience "up" days and "down" days. Enthusiastic supporters spur an ultramarathoner to run a 50-kilometer race faster than he had thought possible. A long-distance swimmer notices that the sensory deprivation of long hours in the ocean causes her to experience hallucinations. Why? Because we're not machines; our minds as well as our bodies affect physical performance. Myriad psychological factors impose limits on athletic accomplishment.

The Inner Game of Endurance

Dissociation. Sports psychologist William P. Morgan has studied the mental states of marathon runners. He has identified a psychological strategy called "dissociation" that helps runners persevere despite pain. Dissociation is a trancelike mental state in which athletes purposely divorce themselves from sensory feedback. Dissociators divert their attention from physical feelings by daydreaming, indulging fantasies, or mumbling repetitious phrases—akin to the mantras used by meditators. They are "lost in space."

Dissociation has both advantages and disadvantages. It can allow athletes to continue despite discomfort or fatigue. But by dulling pain it can also prevent athletes from responding to the warning signs of incipient injury. Existing injuries can be exacerbated by continuing to train or compete when dissociation permits an athlete to ignore pain. At the extreme, the dissociative state could be very hazardous to runners or cyclists training in traffic.

Morgan once had the opportunity to study twenty world-class marathon runners who had assembled at Dr. Kenneth Cooper's Institute for Aerobic Research. He had expected to find that those elite athletes employ a dissociative cognitive strategy. He thought they would be particularly adept at escaping into the ether during a race. To his surprise, Morgan learned that these world-class runners were primarily associators. That is, during races they consciously concentrate on physiological feedback rather than allow themselves to slip into a trance. The top runners monitor their own heart rates and respiration; they stay alert to signs of pain; they try to notice how their joints and limbs feel; and they pay attention to other competitors, the terrain, and scenery.

Despite the practices of these elite runners, dissociation has its beneficial qualities. In an April 1978 *Psychology Today* article entitled "The Mind of the Marathoner," Morgan recommends that endurance athletes temporarily use dissociation to overcome particularly difficult parts of a competition. Thus, a cyclist attacking a hill can slip into a dissociative state during this painful period. Then, after the hill, the cyclist can resume associating. Endurance athletes, who frequently go well beyond the exertion level of a marathon, might have particular use for the ability to go in and out of the dissociative state. On the other hand, an associative strategy would seem essential in order to pace oneself intelligently and have some "juice" left for the finish of an ultradistance event.

Mental Tricks. The ability to deal with motivational crises also imposes a limit on performance. Competitors near the front of the pack are inspired to continue either by the task of staying ahead or by the challenge to catch up, but middle- and back-of-the-pack contestants don't have those incentives. Nonelite athletes must employ other strategies to overcome the temptation to quit during a particularly difficult event. Race participants often report that they employ one of two common mental tricks to break through their performance barriers: the "what next" strategy, or the "never again" strategy.

At midpoint of an ultralong, interisland race in Hawaii a canoeist might say to herself, "I'm halfway done. What's my next event going to be?" By using the what-next trick, the canoeist is able to ignore the fatigue of hours of paddling. Concentrating on the next challenge is a very positive strategy; it implies that the present event will be completed successfully.

A skier named Rob reports that, during the 55-kilometer Birkebeiner, he reached a point at which he felt too tired to go on. Then he fell back on a psychological trick he has used in numerous other events. He told himself, "I don't know why I got myself into this, but I said I would do it, and I will. However, I'll never commit myself to anything like this again." Rob uses the never-again strategy.

Both the what-next and the never-again tricks work to overcome the temptation to quit. Of course, there is nothing wrong with quitting a race when you are injured or ill or just plain bored with it, but most people feel better about completing what they start and would regret not having some defense mechanism that gets them past low points in their morale. Endurance athletes are creative about coming up with techniques to trick themselves into continuing.

Personal Best. Endurance sport's most valuable contribution to society in general may be the concept of the "personal best." Pursuit of individual achievement is another psychological mechanism that permits human performance barriers to be stretched.

The Social Limits

Tangible Incentives.   The second time in 1984 that Yiannis Kouros broke the six-day footrace record, he clearly could have run even farther than he did. He temporarily quit just short of his own record because he was dissatisfied about the prizes. He had not received all the rewards he believed had been promised.

The incentives that are offered to athletes are a major determinant of the achievement limits. Amateurism is fine, but historically, dangling a reward in front of athletes has been the motivation for records to improve. Without prizes, some endurance contests would not occur at all. Without the Kremer prize, Bryan Allen would never have had an opportunity to pedal the *Gossamer Albatross* across the English Channel, because the plane would not have been built in the first place.

Some people fear that money distorts athletics, but elite athletes usually disagree. For years the Western States 100-Miler grew more and more popular among ultradistance runners, largely through word of mouth. Now it has network TV coverage and prize money. Some purists criticize these developments, but the top contestants—who will carry off the modest prizes—say that now they at least will get some reward and recognition for doing what they have done all along.

Behavior Modification.   The social influences to improve athletic performance sometimes operate more subtly than does prize money. Pete Penseyres recounts that during his victorious 1984 Race Across AMerica his handlers noticed that they could make him go faster by playing a psychological trick on him. Chuck Hoefer, his bicycle mechanic, was driving the support vehicle one night and observed that Penseyres had a favorite position in the cone of light provided by the headlamps. Through experimentation Chuck discovered that he could make Penseyres pedal faster by very gradually and imperceptibly increasing the van's speed.

Penseyres was responding to a technique that psychologists call "behavior modification." The technical term for the specific procedure is "shaping." Penseyres's responses were being shaped and manipulated by his desire to keep his bicycle in the best illuminated zone of the road. Used judiciously—and benignly—by coaches and sports psychologists, behavior modification techniques can be another tool to stretch the limits of athletic accomplishment.

Social Facilitation.   Behavior modification is not the only subtle influence to which athletes respond. One of the earliest findings in the field of social psychology was the result of some careful observation of bicycle time trialists. In 1898, N. Triplett, a social psychologist, obtained time-trial statistics from the League of American Wheelmen. Some of the time trialists were riding alone, others were drafting behind tandem bicycles. As might be expected from the substantial aerody- namic advantages of drafting, the paced cyclists went faster than the unpaced cyclists. But some of the *paced* cyclists were timed in indi- vidual heats, while others were timed in groups of two or more *paced* cyclists with each rider drafting off his own team of tandem riders. Those paced cyclists who rode their heats in groups went faster than those who rode their heats individually. Both the individual and the group pacers enjoyed roughly the same opportunity to draft, so Triplett concluded that psychological factors were the only possible explanation for better performance by those who rode in groups.

More than mere competition appears to be involved, because all the cyclists were riding against the clock, not the cyclists who happened to share their heat. In other research, psychologists have discovered that merely thinking that other people are doing the same thing in- creases performance. Apparently we produce more in social settings, and generally that seems to be true for athletics. The psychologists call this phenomenon "social facilitation," because the presence of others seems to facilitate performance.

In endurance athletics social facilitation could have tremendous impact on crashing through the performance barriers. Training with other people and competitive events both offer the possibility of par- ticipating in a social setting, and social facilitation suggests that doing that will make you go faster.

The Guinness Book Phenomenon.   Still another social influence on endurance limits is the keeping of records. Since the late nineteenth century, internationally publicizing records has encouraged athletes to strive just a bit harder. The incentive of a record has pushed elite athletes to new heights. Lesser athletes are also influenced by the record books, because absolute standards allow them to gauge their performance on a worldwide basis. If you live in a community where few people practice your sport, you can *only* evaluate how good you are by looking to the record books.

Records have a tendency to pull athletes to new levels of perfor- mance. In July 1985, shortly after she ran a 2:21.06 marathon, which lowered the women's record by more than a minute and a half, Ingrid Kristiansen told *Runner's World,* "The world record for men is 2:07.11. And so 2:20 is not a very good time for men, but for women, yes, 2:20 is a very good time. And why is that? Because nobody has done it before." Kristiansen had set her sights on 2:20 while she still was basking in the glow of her new world record.

The existence of a recognized record occasionally is the only in- centive for people to pursue a sport at all. When John Marino gained notoriety by establishing a record for crossing the United States by bicycle, it inspired Lon Haldeman to challenge his record. Haldeman might have accomplished other things as an endurance cyclist, but he probably wouldn't have pushed back that particular performance barrier if the record had not been there to break. Initially, the cross-continental record attempts were solo affairs, but the existence of a recognized record ultimately led to head-to-head competition, and that in turn decreased the crossing time by four days over a period of just seven years.

The Self-fulfilling Prophecy

Psychologist Robert Rosenthal has suggested a theory that may explain the most formidable limit to endurance. He believes that humans often respond to self-fulfilling prophecies. That is, they cannot exceed the performance that they themselves or other people predict for them.

The self-fulfilling prophecy, or SFP, is more than a superstitious notion, because it operates on several nonmagical levels. For instance, people who do not believe they can swim across the lake are not likely to dive into the water in the first place. Hence, their SFP's will automatically be correct, because they in fact did not swim across the lake. Similarly, if I am near my automobile at mile 23 of my first marathon, and I don't believe I can make it to the finish line soon enough to win a T-shirt, I might as well quit where I am, rather than run 3 more miles and then need to walk 3 miles back to my car. Again, my prophecy came true.

Bryan Allen's physiologist, Joseph Mastropaolo, once told him something related to the SFP that possibly made the crucial difference in his successful human-powered flight across the English Channel. (Aside from his scientific credentials as a physiologist, Mastropaolo is also a graduate of the École Supérieure D'Escrime, a prestigious and exclusive fencing academy in Paris. Mastropaolo attained championship level in his weapon, the épée.) Allen recounts the advice: "One of Mastropaolo's fencing masters beat into his head, and he beat into mine, that the difference between winning and losing was just internal volition. It's a pretty powerful concept. Once you get to the pinnacle of athletic achievement, the difference between winning and losing is just who has the strongest volition. The ability to look around at all the other competitors and say, 'Why did all these people show up today if the best they can get is second place?' And really believing that too, not doing that as some sort of egotistical statement, but as a realized fact: 'Wow, everybody else is going to get second. Why'd they even show up?' That was really important on the cross-Channel flight because the biggest competitor we had was the unknown. This was something nobody had even come close to doing."

The self-fulfilling prophecy may be the final frontier of endurance.

INDIVIDUAL AND GROUP DIFFERENCES

WHAT makes an athlete?

Probably all of us at some time or other have asked that question. If we'd been born with Scott Tinley's legs, or were ten years younger, or had more slow-twitch muscle fibers, or had trained since we were twelve, could we have won the Ironman?

The answer is still being debated by researchers in sports medicine, psychology, and other fields. Nobody knows.

It all goes back to the old argument of nature versus nurture, touched upon in the previous chapter. We're still trying to sort out how much of what we are is inherited, and how much comes from our environment. (There's actually a third element of the equation, but more on that later.)

We got our genetic makeup the moment we were conceived, and scientists are still trying to figure out what it consists of. We know our genes determine what sex we are and what we look like, what color our hair, eyes, and skin are, and whether we have a nose like Grandfather Herman's or Aunt Sarah's. We also know genes determine our height and weight. But here matters start to get a little fuzzy. Height and weight are also influenced by environment—whether your mother practiced proper nutrition when she was pregnant with you, and whether you grew up with a balanced diet and enough exercise.

About fifteen years ago, researchers started finding out that our genes not only determine the way we look, but they also play a role in the way we behave. That's when things started to get complicated. We all know, for instance, that our environment determines how intelligent we will become. If you doubt it, just listen to the commercials for home computers and educational software. Today, however, there is evidence that the upper limits of our intellectual abilities—just how bright it is possible for us to become if we work at it and have every advantage—are set by our genes and that a four-foot stack of floppy disks won't get us beyond that maximal point.

There is also mounting evidence that our physical potential is determined in the same way. The good news is that's only the maximal level, *the very most you can do*. How well you perform up to that point appears to be largely up to you.

Recently, physiological profiles were run on two champion ultramarathoners. One, thirty-year-old Barney Klecker, was the world record holder at 50 miles (4:51.25). The other, Ben "Chick" Mostow, holds the 50-mile record (10:22.43) for the seventy-five-years-and-over age group. Mostow is seventy-eight.

The results of the study showed that both men had physiological characteristics that were similar to those of other marathoners and ultramarathoners, but surprisingly, the researchers found no inherited characteristics that would account for their superiority over other athletes. They are elite athletes, but they are not genetically elite!

So don't pack away your Nikes just because no one in your family ever won any races. If you do, you're reckoning without the nurture part of the equation. That's your environment—and it may include a lot more than you think.

Your environment starts to exert its influence over you as soon as you are conceived. Our first environment is our mother's womb, and researchers are finding out today that a lot more goes on there than we'd ever before imagined. The illnesses and stresses your mother might have experienced before you were born could have affected your developing nervous system. The foods she ate contributed directly to your own nutritional development. Mothers who use tobacco, alcohol, and various other drugs during pregnancy expose the fetus to the risk of premature birth and generally have smaller, less intelligent children than mothers who don't use those drugs. We also have evidence now that a developing fetus can perceive sunlight and hear sounds. Some parents even have begun to make a practice of singing to, playing music for, or talking to their unborn children.

Once we're born, *other people* enter our environment—family, friends, teachers, faces from the TV screen. That's when the fun begins. These people, along with the nation and city or town we live in, the school we go to, our neighborhood, the books and magazines we read, the TV programs we watch, all go to make up our culture, which is our environment, too. Its effect on us is profound. No one yet has determined the full extent of cultural influence.

We know that cultural factors play an enormous role in athletics, in determining who chooses what sport, but sometimes it's hard to determine where genetic influences leave off and cultural influences begin. The fact that there now are so many black sprinters and so few black endurance athletes is one example. It is commonly believed that blacks are well equipped genetically for short distances and less well equipped for long distances. But one striking physiological trait common to blacks makes them supremely suitable for endurance events: they carry less body fat than whites or Orientals.

Lately, several fine black distance runners have made news, and today more blacks are participating in distance events and performing better in them overall than before. During the past decade numerous black runners from Kenya, such as Henry Rono, have done extremely well in long-distance events. So far, the only athlete of any race to win two Olympic marathons is the late Abebe Bikila of Ethiopia. Way back in 1880, the six-day record was held for a time by a black ultra-marathoner, Frank Hart, who walked and ran 565 miles to win a "go as you please" race at Madison Square Garden. Now there are few black ultradistance runners, but notable exceptions to the stereotype make their relative absence in the marathon lineups appear more due to cultural factors than to any genetic traits that make them exceptional sprinters but lackluster distance runners.

Some deep-seated cultural factors discourage long-distance running by black Americans. Fear of racial violence is one of them. A few years ago, Norm Chambers, a black psychologist in Southern California whose son had quarterbacked his high school football team to an undefeated season, explained it this way: "I'm not so sure I want Eric out there running. Some cop is liable to kill him because he assumes that any young black man running on the street must be fleeing a crime. Eric's just the right age, too."

Although one of the earliest American sports heroes of any race, in any sport, was a turn-of-the-century black bicycle road racer by the name of Major Taylor, few blacks have excelled at cycling since then. More recently, at the 1984 Olympic Games a black sprinter, Nelson Vails, became one of the first Americans to win an Olympic medal for cycling since the 1912 Games.

This makes the shortage of black cyclists also seem more determined by cultural factors than genes. To get an idea of how powerful an influence social and cultural factors can be, we need only look back at how few black tennis players there were before Arthur Ashe came on the scene.

Despite the enormous role our environment plays in our athletic development, the most crucial factor in our physical prowess is clearly genetically determined. That is our sex.

Men are larger than women. They also carry less body fat. Those two factors give them an enormous advantage over women in some sports.

The most obvious difference between men and women—and probably the one we think least about—is body size. The average height for women between the ages of twenty and twenty-four is 64.5 inches. For men of the same age it's 68.5 inches. Round those figures off to 65 and 69 inches and check the U.S. Public Health and Nutrition Survey for average weights. You'll find a five-foot-five woman averages 149 pounds between ages eighteen and seventy-four, and a five-foot-nine man averages 173.

The differences in height occur because the female hormone estrogen stops a woman's growth about two years earlier than growth stops in men. But even when men and women of identical heights are compared, the men are heavier. The average five-foot-five man weighs 155 pounds and a five-foot-nine woman weighs only 158.

This range of height and weight seems to hold true for athletes as well as the rest of the population, despite the effect physical activity has on body weight.

A man's larger body size typically gives him larger internal organs, also. This means that his lungs require and are capable of processing more oxygen than a woman's lungs, giving him greater aerobic capacity. It also means a heart 10 to 20 percent larger than that of a woman—which means a heart that pumps more blood. Males' larger body size also means they have more blood to pump—12 to 25 percent more than females. This, too, contributes to better aerobic capacity.

(Women apparently compensate somewhat for their smaller hearts by maintaining a heart rate at rest and during light activity that's greater than a man's heart rate when he's doing the same things. But since the maximal heart rate of both sexes is about the same, men still chalk up a 30 percent greater maximal cardiac output.)

This does *not* mean all women are inferior to all men in performing physical tasks. Many women are better athletes than a large number of men. What these studies *do* show is that if men and women are paired in terms of height and relative weight, age, training, and other factors, statistically the men will outperform the women. The reasons are the male's greater size and, as we shall see, the female's larger proportion of body fat.

The average woman carries 10 to 15 pounds more adipose tissue on her frame than the average man. His lean body mass is about 12 to 16 percent. Hers is 22 to 26 percent. This handicaps a woman's athletic performance in two ways. First, she has less muscle mass to exert the force that will give her speed, power, strength, and endurance. Second, she has to perform while carrying an extra 10 to 15 pounds of dead weight, her extra fatty tissue.

"Enough, already. I'll diet," you might say.

Well, some of that fat is essential. And the men have got you beat there, too.

Researchers believe that the average man carries about 3 percent essential fat plus 12 percent storage fat. The average woman, however, carries about 12 percent essential fat and 15 percent storage fat.

What makes essential fat so essential?

Scientists believe essential fat is necessary for the body to function properly. It's in your heart, kidneys, intestines, liver, lungs, central nervous system, and bone marrow. In women it includes fatty tissue in the breasts and possibly the thighs and pelvic region.

Now that the female readers are thoroughly discouraged, here comes the good part. Nurture.

The figures above were for *average* men and women, who tend to be a lot more sedentary than endurance athletes. Some women distance runners have trained down to 6 percent body fat and suffered no apparent ill effects. So both nature and nurture have a role in body composition.

One theory maintains that a woman's additional body fat can actually benefit her in endurance events. Dr. Joan Ullyot wrote in 1976 that women were the perfect long-distance runners because they are not slowed down by heavy musculature, they carry an abundance of fat for fuel, and they can burn their fat more effectively than men. Unfortunately for women, however, this hypothesis has not been borne out in preliminary testing. When men and women were tested after a sixty-mile treadmill run at 70 percent of the maximum aerobic power, the women did not process their fat any more effectively than the men.

In running and cycling you carry your body weight, and dead weight will slow you down. In swimming, it's a different story. Fatty tissue can come in handy for helping you stay afloat. Women swimmers carry 18 to 22 percent body fat. In open-water swimming, fat also protects you against hypothermia. Gertrude Ederle, Grete Anderson, and Diana Nyad have beaten all or most of their male competitors in long-distance open-water swim races.

Human muscle fibers have been divided by scientists into two categories, slow-twitch and fast-twitch, according to the way they contract and the way they burn fuel. Men and women seem to have about an equal percentage of each. The percentages vary significantly with the type of sport a person plays, however. Sprinters and power athletes have a higher percentage of fast-twitch fibers and endurance athletes have a higher percentage of slow-twitch fibers. This holds true for both sexes.

In spite of the fact that their muscle composition is similar, the average man shows up in studies about 30 to 40 percent stronger than the average woman. The biggest difference is in upper-body strength. The smallest difference is in the legs.

When women train, however, they can increase their strength in short order. Women in one study, after just ten weeks of training, had attained the leg strength of untrained men.

There is nothing we can do but accept our biological differences. Differences that result from our behavior, however, can readily be changed. Women respond the same ways men do to exercise and training. That is, after training, they can go farther faster and get there in better physiological condition than they could before.

It is no accident that older athletes choose to do endurance activities. Distance runners and cyclists have their best years relatively late, compared to participants in other sports. At thirty-seven, Carlos Lopes of Portugal won the 1984 Olympic marathon, and then in 1985 set a world record (2:07.11) for the same distance. Peter Penseyres waited until he was forty-two years old to set the transcontinental bicycle record and win the 1984 Race Across AMerica. (For endurance swimmers the peak is roughly fifteen years earlier, late teens to early twenties.)

The legions of men and women who work out their midlife crises by training for marathons are all mere children compared to growing numbers of older competitors.

Eighty-year-old Ruth Goldfarb ran the 1982 Avon Half-Marathon in New York.

The "great American pedestrian," Edward Payson Weston, continued to accomplish highly publicized long-distance walks well into his seventies. As a spry seventy-four-year-old, he completed his last major walk, a mere 1,500-mile perambulation, from New York City to Minneapolis.

In 1984, fifty-four-year-old Sister Marion Irvine became the oldest person to qualify for the U.S. Olympic marathon trials. Her 2:51.01 performance in the California International Marathon was the equivalent of an over-fifty man running 2:18, which is ten minutes faster than any man that age has ever run.

Annabel Marsh, sixty-one, and Caroline Merrill, forty-two, ran across the United States in 1984.

In his late seventies, Walt Stack of San Francisco does ultramarathons, and at seventy-six he completed the Ironman Triathlon.

The truly amazing thing about all this is that every year such feats by older people become less amazing. Participation in masters competitions has burgeoned in recent years. Virtually every major endurance competition has a category for the over-sixty crowd and sometimes even over-seventy entrants.

Although even the best athlete's prowess starts to decline slowly around age forty, it's no surprise that training for endurance compe-

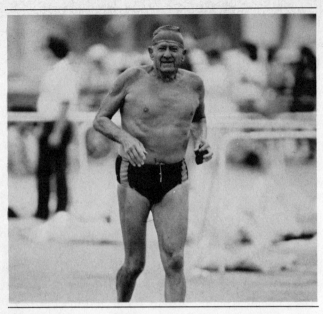

Al Guth, in his mid-seventies, finishes the swim at the Los Angeles USTS Triathlon. PHOTO BY BUDD SYMES

tition seems to retard the aging process. *Competition* is the key word here. Twenty-four regional and national track champions were followed in a ten-year study. At the time of the study the athletes ranged in age from fifty to eighty-two. They were all still running, and at almost the same distances, but only eleven were training intensely and competing. These eleven showed less of a reduction in such important characteristics as aerobic capacity, percentage of body fat, and lean body weight than the group who had quit competing but continued to run.

If you do continue to train hard and compete into your fifties, sixties, and seventies, it's beginning to look as if the benefits could be enormous. Recently, researchers compared two female masters swimmers, aged seventy and seventy-one, with sedentary women of the same age and with younger female athletes. Both women were members of the 1980 All-American Masters Swim Team. They turned out to have a considerably lower percentage of body fat than normal sedentary women in their seventies and were well within the range for normal women nineteen to twenty-five years old. Their aerobic capacity was approximately twice that for the average female in her seventies and comparable to female nonathletes who were considerably younger.

Expanded interest in masters swimming competition for women is attracting a growing number of participants who are fifty and above.

It's easy to see why. The seventy- and seventy-one-year-old women in the study had body-fat percentages equal to college-age women in the sports of tennis and shotput and discus throwing and the aerobic capacity of sedentary women who were twenty years old!

Nature and nurture work together to make us what we are. The genes we inherit are not grim biological determinants. Neither are they a guarantee of a shelf full of trophies.

And now the third part of the nature-nuture equation. That's us. The decisions we make. How we use what we're born with and the things we take from our environment around us to become what we are.

Look again at the fast-twitch and slow-twitch muscle differences between sprinters and distance runners for one illustration of the importance of choice in athletics. Muscle composition appears to be genetically set. Training alters it very little. The high percentage of fast-twitch muscle fibers in top sprinters and slow-twitch fibers in top distance runners is therefore almost entirely the result of choice. We choose to take a sport seriously enough to compete in it if we show early promise for it.

You'll never win a triathlon if you don't train. That's another athletic choice to make. If you do decide to train, even to the best of your ability, the odds are that you will not become a champion. That's mostly nature, and only a few of us have championship genes. But whatever your age or sex, you can train hard and rack up a proud personal best in a chosen sport—if you decide to.

TO THE BRINK OF DEATH

IN THE 1981 Ironman, Teiichiro Tsutsumi, a fifty-six-year-old Japanese surgeon, finished next to last. He swam the backstroke guided by a mirror mounted on his chest for over five hours in order to complete just the first segment. The entire event took him over twenty-five hours. At the post-triathlon banquet he won a crying towel for his efforts. (The man he beat, seventy-six-year-old Walt Stack, had already won a prize for the oldest finisher.)

It was not Dr. Tsutsumi's athletic prowess that has lived in the hearts and minds of his fellow competitors, but his eloquent summation of the event. After accepting his award, he struggled bravely to express his thanks in halting English peppered with such recognizable but unconnected phrases as "want water" and "tired." But he went straight to the heart of the matter—and won tumultuous applause—when he ended his speech by blurting out, "Almos' *die!*"

His words were a figure of speech, of course. But there's an element of truth in them. The risk of injury or death is present in all sports, but it is particularly great in endurance athletics because the events are so challenging. Part of the challenge is that we do not even know what the limits of human endurance are.

In the Western States 100-Miler some runners have exerted until they collapsed from exhaustion, despite medical safeguards. Ultra-distance runner Alex Lievanos reached the Robinson Flats aid station at mile 32 of the Western States and was told by the doctors, "You've got no blood pressure, we're yanking you out." With liquids and food Lievanos managed to revive himself sufficiently to obtain the doctors' grudging permission to proceed. He lasted another 8 miles and then fell down on the trail. He could go no farther, but he lived to tell the tale.

Tenacity is commonplace for endurance athletes. The athletes generally have invested too much training to quit because of early adversity. Triathlete Paul Bush completed his first Ironman despite severe jelly-fish stings he sustained during the swim. T. J. Key once

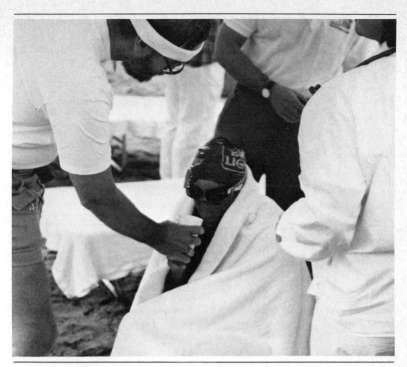

A hypothermia victim after the swim at the San Diego USTS race.   PHOTO BY ALBERT GROSS

collapsed during an ultramarathon, slept it off, got up, resumed running, and went on to win the race—because he was the only finisher. The resolve of endurance athletes is laudable, but occasionally their willingness to persevere in the face of hazards calls the entire enterprise into question.

"The most serious risk you take is death," Robert Lind, a physician for the rugged Western States 100-Miler, once told a reporter. Lind says that runners experience nausea, vomiting, headaches, dizziness, irritability, lassitude, weakness, pounding pulse, hallucinations, paranoia—all symptoms of dehydration, hypothermia, hypoglycemia, and renal failure.

When you consider the rigorous demands ultrasports make on the human body, it's surprising that mishaps are as few as they are. Statistics show that most people taking part in endurance events are not overdoing it. In 1984, 16,315 people started the New York City Marathon and 89.4 percent finished.

The sheer difficulty of endurance events has a lot to do with their safety. People respect them and train for them seriously. A person who is untrained and out of shape may take up a challenge in a bar one night and go out and tackle an ultramarathon the next day. But fatigue will usually put a stop to that foolishness before too much damage is done.

The flip side of endurance sports is that the positive-thinking "I can do it" attitude they demand can lead a trained athlete to treat lightly warning signals that shouldn't be ignored.

The 1982 Ironman was Julie Moss's first. She was trained, but inexperienced. She fell victim to exhaustion, lost control of her bodily functions, and dragged herself the last 15 feet across the finish line to take the women's second place in what has become the most publicized wipeout in endurance sports.

"I didn't suffer from heat stroke in the race," she told *The New York Times* the following year. "I was lucid. I ran out of food, and my legs got rubbery. If I was 3 miles from the finish, I would have pulled over and rested. But I was so close. I was thinking, 'Why do you have to fall down in front of an ABC camera?' " She added that, despite her collapse, "I was nowhere near dying." Two years later she told a *Triathlon* magazine interviewer that she should have walked that final mile.

Conrad Will, on the other hand, was a seasoned triathlete when he organized the 1984 Big Island Triathlon in Kona. This was a three-day, three-stage meet. Participants swam 6 miles, bicycled 235 miles around the Big Island of Hawaii, and ran 52.4 miles on the final day.

The swim and 65 miles of bicycling comprised the first day. That left 170 bicycle miles for day two. When Will finished the second day's ride, he sat down to rest at the finish line and began trembling violently. His support crew rushed him to a nearby hospital, where he was given intravenous fluid for severe dehydration and hypoglycemia. "If he had waited just five more minutes or had gone to sleep he could have gone into shock," said the emergency physician who treated him. "Very severe consequences could have resulted."

Elite distance runner Alberto Salazar's brushes with disaster have given him the longest thermometer in professional sports. In August 1978 the 7.1 miles of the Falmouth Road Race were packed with some four thousand overheated runners. The humidity got to veteran runner Bill Rodgers, who had the lead at 4.5 miles. "I couldn't surge anymore," he said later. "I knew I wasn't going to win."

He was wrong.

Salazar, running a half step behind and feeling like he could fry an egg on his own forehead, drew alongside Rodgers and said, "Bill, you've been doing the work. Why don't I take over?" Rodgers turned to tell him, "It's your race," but when he looked around, Salazar had fallen ten yards behind.

A mile and a half from the finish, Alberto Salazar really began to fade. "Everything went out of me," he told *Sports Illustrated*. "The world looked strange. It was fuzzy and had dim patches. People passed me, four or five in the last half mile. I can't remember anything after the finish. I woke up in a bathtub full of ice.''

His temperature had soared briefly to 108 degrees. Doctors administered intravenous saline solution and he returned to normal quickly, then passed on to subnormal in his icy bath. "They cooled me off in the ice, right down to 94 degrees," he said, "then they had to get me warm again.''

Ninety-four turned out to be nowhere as low as Salazar could go. Four years later, appearing exhausted to the point of pain, he won the Boston Marathon by a scant two seconds and ten yards. Salazar stayed on his feet long enough to receive the laurel crown. Then he collapsed.

His problem this time was the opposite of what had happened at Falmouth: his temperature had plummeted to 88 degrees. He was suffering this time not from heat stroke but from heat exhaustion. His skin was cold and clammy, and Dr. Thomas F. O'Donnel, Jr., from Tufts New England Medical Center, pronounced him dehydrated "as a potato chip.''

How could running a marathon cool his body so?

Running generates heat and the body sweats so it can cool itself through evaporation. A well-conditioned runner can lose more than 1.5 quarts of fluid an hour. The weather in Falmouth had been hot and humid, but the heat in Boston was dry with a good steady breeze. That dry breeze made the difference. It aided evaporation and Salazar cooled rapidly. When the race was over, he kept on cooling. Since he was no longer running to generate heat, his temperature dipped dramatically and he collapsed.

Because he got proper and immediate medical treatment, he was actually in little danger. Doctors wrapped him in blankets and Mylar foil to warm his body and gave him intravenous saline solution and glucose. Although his temperature registered 88 on an oral thermometer, internally it was probably higher. Through it all, his blood pressure remained normal, which meant he was in little danger of going into shock.

How could Salazar have become so dehydrated without realizing it? How could Julie Moss have run out of fuel so suddenly in the Ironman? Perhaps the answer lies in the euphoria long-distance exertion produces.

Even though we may not have experienced it, we've all heard of the "runner's high.'' A similar effect occurs in other endurance sports. Long-distance swimmer Diana Nyad listed the four stages in a marathon swim for *Psychology Today* as "hurt, pain, agony, and pleasure, in that order.''

Her testimony was seconded by Cindy Erlish, a San Francisco

writer who did the Escape from Alcatraz Swim: "You do get images when you're in the water that long, and you lose your sense of time. There is a lot of pain at first, but if you go through it you get to a kind of euphoria, and when the swim is over you don't want to come out of the water."

How else but on a runner's high could Dennis Rainier have finished a marathon in three hours and nine minutes *when he ran the last 16 miles with a .22 caliber slug in his skull?*

Yes, you read that right. In 1978 Rainier was running a marathon in Allendale, Michigan, trying for the three-hour finish that would qualify him for the Boston Marathon. Near the 10-mile mark, he said "something that felt about the size of a brick" hit his head. Thinking it was a rock thrown up by a passing car, he kept on running. Only after the race was over did he find out he'd been hit by a bullet! (Despite the fact that his time was nine minutes over the qualifying mark, Rainier got to run in Boston. Marathon officials gave him a special invitation.)

There's evidence that endurance euphoria can distort perceptions even in suffering. Julie Moss had no sense of the slowness of her agonizing crawl to the Ironman finish. "I thought I was really speeding along," she told a reporter later. "I just wanted to keep crawling through everybody's legs, cross the line and get a shower."

Sensory and sleep deprivation are two other conditions that can play havoc with the safety of endurance sports.

Diana Nyad described for *Psychology Today* the effect of sensory deprivation in a marathon swim: "You drop into a hypnotic trance. It's not only that you're doing something for eight or 10 or 20 hours, but also your communication is cut off. I wear tight rubber caps on my ears; I can't hear very well at all. The goggles just fit over my eyes and I'm turning my head 60 times every minute, so I don't see very much.

"I don't have time in that eighth of a second that the breath lasts to focus on anything. A lot of childhood and sexual images go through my mind—quick, dreamlike flashes that come like a picture on a movie screen. When I've finished a swim I feel like I know myself better."

Enlightenment is certainly a desirable thing, but such a narrowed and inward focus can be dangerous in some endurance situations. Think of a cyclist dodging cars on the open roads.

Another potentially dangerous condition that accompanies the longer ultrasports is sleep deprivation. If you go without sleep long enough, dreams begin to intrude on your waking state, producing hallucinations and, in some cases, even paranoia.

John Howard pedaled virtually nonstop for ten days against John

Marino, Lon Haldeman, and Michael Shermer in the Great American Bike Race from Santa Monica Pier to the Empire State Building in 1982. After falling behind due to illness on the first day, he pushed himself to catch up through the rest of the race. The following is his vivid description of the weird visions that kept him company on his trek:

"All through Arizona and New Mexico I had one recurring hallucination that was different from the others. The first one, a clump of trees that appeared to be a man on a horse, was the simplest of all my visions, being merely an optical illusion that involved no motion or other attributes. Other later apparitions were more mobile and animated, but still they were primarily visual phenomena. But in a class by itself was my Great Southwest Hallucination. It was *physical* as well as visual, and it was very powerful.

"Imagine riding mile after mile, hour after hour, under an enormous sky, with very little else to see but the horizon and the road. Then imagine that sky as a wall or a ceiling that presses steadily down, narrowing all the while the amount of space there is to ride in. Now imagine the pressing to be physical and visual at the same time, making *you* heavy and sluggish, pressing you to the ground, flattening you like putty under a steam roller.

"That is what I lived and rode under through most of Arizona, all of New Mexico, little chips of Texas and Oklahoma, and the greater part of Kansas—a good one-third of the distance across the country, 1,000 miles under pressure. Over and over this enormous gray press would trap me, pressing, oppressing, depressing me, and slowing me down, seemingly to a crawl. No doubt the constant head winds and the vast horizon contributed to the forcefulness of this hallucination.

"I could dispel it by blinking hard and shaking my head, but it would return. My only defense was to play with the hallucination, look forward to it, let it wash over me and massage me. And that is what I did."

Not all Howard's visions on the trip were oppressive and grim. One morning outside Wichita he was pedaling along alone and hungry, the motor home that carried his support team temporarily out of sight. Suddenly he saw Sandy Daggett, the woman who was his nurse and cook, standing a little ways ahead in the road, wearing a white dress that billowed in the wind and holding out her hand as if proffering something to eat. "She was such a refreshing sight that her image sustained me until the crew finally found me and gave me some more substantial nourishment," Howard later recalled.

Another hallucination, however, carried a strong potential for danger. It came to the cyclist many times, always at night. "The pavement ahead of me would come alive to become multidirectional and complicated, rather than just a plain roadway," Howard remembers. "Like some three-dimensional Escher print, there would appear before me a complex series of ramps going in all directions. I would have to choose one to ride on, and it would seem to be an opening in the pavement that both had no end and yet narrowed to a point.

"I would seem to descend below the level of the road—in fact, I could see the layers of materials that comprised the highway, from the surface asphalt down to the underlying boulders and rubble—and just as I reached the point where the sky was no longer visible, the hallucination would quit."

One night, when the ramps appeared, Howard said he "could feel one path beckoning me; it seemed to call me by name. I followed it until the honking of my support vehicle brought me to my senses." The "ramp" he had taken on that occasion turned out to be an intersecting country road identified by a sign as "Howard Road."

The cyclist's last truly memorable hallucination occurred one night in the mountains of West Virginia. The weather was cold and foggy and he had stopped to answer a call of nature. "I saw a dog, a pretty combination Irish setter and Labrador retriever, much like a dog I know," Howard recalled. "It was there wagging its tail and smiling as only a setter can do; then it was lying down; then it was decayed and long dead. These visions were like snapshots: one, two, three. Only they were in three dimensions, holographs from my mind. I can only guess what they meant. I was about as loony as I ever expect to be."

By far the most serious threat born of sleep deprivation, as competitors in the Great American Bike Race found out, is not hallucinations but being overtaken by sleep. "One moment I am pedaling normally; the next instant my legs have locked up and I've lost my balance. The ensuing swerving, waking, and righting is instantaneous and chilling," says Howard. Fellow GABR cyclist Michael Shermer fell asleep on his bike and hit a guard rail. He escaped unharmed, but the bike was ruined. In the 1984 Race Across AMerica (the descendant of the GABR) Lon Haldeman hit the pavement several times.

The dangers posed by sleep deprivation on the Great American Bike Race led Howard to conclude later that "any one of us could have gone down in front of a truck or over a cliff for a permanent snooze." He recommended any future runnings of the GABR include a mandatory three-hour rest period, preferably sometime during the night, every twenty-four hours.

The environment of some endurance contests automatically provides the danger. Drowning is always a possibility on marathon swims; more than one swimmer has been pulled from the water unconscious, the victim of hypothermia or exhaustion. On February 5, 1927, Myrtle

Huddlestone became the frst woman to swim across the 21-mile channel between Catalina Island and the California coast. However, she had to recuperate from her swim (20:42) in the hospital. She was not just exhausted, she had also been slashed and bitten by barracudas during the swim. During her double crossing of the Catalina Channel in 1977, Cindy Cleveland was harassed by a shark until the navigator of her support boat gaffed the animal. "Just when you thought it was safe to go back in the water . . ."

Sometimes dangers arise in ultrasports due to unforeseen conditions surrounding the events.

Although they were not, strictly speaking, undertaken for sport, the early Arctic and Antarctic expeditions—preairplane, prehelicopter, and presnowmobile—were certainly extreme tests of participants' endurance. One in particular, that of a group of British explorers led by Robert F. Scott, is a sobering example of the havoc the elements can wreak on even the most carefully made plans. It is also an illustration of extreme courage in the face of death.

Scott, an officer in the British navy, had been selected in 1900 to command the first National Antarctic Expedition. Everything that time had gone extremely well. With his closest friend, Dr. Edward A. Wilson, and Lieutenant Ernest H. Shakleton, he had discovered Antarctica's Great Ice Barrier and brought back much useful scientific information.

In 1909, Scott organized another expedition. His party of thirty-two included six officers and twelve scientists, one of whom was his friend Dr. Wilson. The group landed in January 1911, near Scott's former base on McMurdo Sound.

They spent the first year making exploratory journeys and established a large depot, which they called "One-Ton Depot," 130 miles from their base camp on a route toward the South Pole.

In late October 1911, Scott and eleven others set out for the Pole. They took motorized sledges, ponies, and dog teams. The sleds soon broke down. The ponies had to be shot before they reached Beardmore Glacier, their most formidable terrain barrier. On December 10, they began to ascend the glacier, pulling three sledges themselves. By December 31, seven men and all the dog teams had to be sent back to the camp.

Scott, Wilson, and the three men continued and reached the South Pole on January 17, 1912, after an exhausting eighty-one-day trek. To their bitter disappointment, they discovered that Roald Amundsen's Norwegian exploration party had beaten them there by about a month. (Unlike Scott's, Amundsen's successful expedition had employed dog teams all the way to the Pole and back.)

The disheartened men were plagued by bad weather on their

return journey. One, Edgar Evans, collapsed and died at the foot of Beardmore Glacier on February 17. Another, L.E.G. Oates, suffering from severe frostbite and feeling himself a burden to the others, crawled out into a blizzard to die on March 17.

The three survivors struggled on for another 10 miles before a nine-day blizzard confined them to their tent. With quiet fortitude they awaited their deaths—only 11 miles from the safety of One-Ton Depot, their destination.

On March 29, Scott wrote the final entry in the diary he had scrupulously kept through the entire expedition: "Every day we have been ready to start for our depot *11 miles* away, but outside the door of the tent it remains a scene of whirling drift. . . . We shall stick it out to the end, but we are getting weaker, of course, and the end cannot be far. It seems a pity, but I do not think I can write more."

On November 12, 1912, searchers found the tent and the three frozen bodies, along with Scott's records and diaries and geological specimens from Beardmore.

The Scott expedition is admittedly an extreme example of adverse conditions. As yet, there is no Snowman Triathlon in Antarctica. Some believe, however, that for sheer enormity the Great American Bike Race and its successor, the Race Across AMerica, closely approximate such an event.

Take, for example, John Howard's experience in that race. He was trying to catch up with Lon Haldeman, who had taken the lead very early in the race and kept it. The desert heat that plagued the GABR cyclists on the first day was incredible—temperatures as high as 112 degrees by 5:00 P.M. and 115 by 6:30! Shortly after dark, Howard's muscles began to cramp. By the time he hit the Arizona border, around 11:00 P.M., he climbed off his bike and sought shelter in the motor home, so cramped and delirious he was unable to continue. He took potassium tablets, recommended by his doctor to alleviate the pain, but they did no good.

"I still don't know what went wrong," recalls Howard. "The problems initially started when I chased Haldeman down after hitting a red light sometime in the late afternoon. It was a good couple of minutes before the light turned green, and I had to sprint a long way to catch up with him. I must have looked bad, because the crew called the doctor right away. Anyway, by midnight I was finished. I went to sleep right there on the Arizona border. By the time I woke up it was light out. I was in last place and only marginally better than the night before."

The race log for day two notes that "Howard, suffering from severe muscle spasms, had slept at the California/Arizona border for more than five hours."

The referee's report, according to the race log, indicated that the cyclist looked and felt "wasted." The referee expressed doubt that his condition would permit him to finish the race. He recommended Howard undergo an immediate physical examination, since he appeared to be suffering from heat prostration.

Howard's pulse was the only thing that kept him in the GABR. It was around 60, instead of the 98 his doctor had expected to find. So Howard pressed on, forcing himself to eat and to get on his bike and ride. "I realized that I'd have to ride this race basically nonstop or pack it in," he said later. "I'd had my last serious sleep." And so he rode onward and into hallucinations.

Even training for an endurance event can be fraught with peril. In a stretch of the San Gabriel Mountains just north of Pasadena, runners training for the Western States 100-Miler and similar rugged ultramarathons may run as much as 50 miles a day at altitudes ranging from 5,000 to 7,000 feet.

In January 1985, forty-nine-year-old runner Herman Kuhn, a "regular" in the San Gabriels, fell 1,900 feet to his death. Park officials had warned him on that windy Saturday against taking a treacherous icy trail that runs past the Mount Wilson Observatory. It was a warning Kuhn did not heed.

Bill Johnson, who owns a running equipment store, also trains in the San Gabriel Mountains. One day he and his running buddies came upon a strange-looking religious ceremony in an isolated location. A number of people dressed in robes were chanting, "Sacrifice." As Johnson told the *Los Angeles Times,* "I was the slowest runner of the group, but I was blazing a path from that."

As both San Gabriel incidents illustrate, arduous endurance training is a lot safer when you don't undertake it alone.

Besides using the buddy system, most endurance athletes learn other means to avoid the substantial risks of their sports. Experienced athletes generally heed the warnings of pain and back off so they will be able to train or compete another day. They know to use proper equipment, and they usually respect the dangers posed by weather, terrain, the elements, and fatigue.

Still, endurance athletes are occasionally injured or killed by their activities. If the events were neither dangerous nor difficult they wouldn't be endurance events. Endurance athletes occasionally teeter on the brink of death, but they are no more suicidal than any other segment of the population. In fact, endurance athletes celebrate life and human spirit by accomplishing the most difficult physical feats they can imagine. They endure.

RECOMMENDED READING

BOOKS

Ahluwalia, Bholi. *Faces of Everest*. New Delhi, India: Vikas Publishing House, 1978.
Narrative (with photos) of Everest assaults.

Caldwell, John. *The Cross-Country Ski Book* (sixth edition). Brattleboro, Vermont: Stephen Greene Press, 1981.
Equipment, participants, technique, and ambience of cross-country skiing.

Cordellos, Harry. *Breaking Through*. Mountain View, California: Anderson World, 1981.
The autobiography of a versatile endurance athlete who is blind.

Cumming, John. *Runners and Walkers*. Chicago: Regnery Gateway, 1981.
A detailed, yet entertaining, account of the history of running during the nineteenth and early twentieth centuries. Illustrated with numerous historical photos and engravings.

Dean, Penny. *How to Swim a Marathon*. Colorado Springs, Colorado: United States Swimming, 1984.
A no-nonsense guide on how to train for endurance swimming.

Foley, Vernard, and Werner, Soedell. "Ancient Oared Warships." *Scientific American,* April 1981, 148–63.
History and technology of classical oared war galleys.

Gross, Albert, Chester Kyle and Douglas Malewicki. "The Aerodynamics of Human-Powered Land Vehicles." *Scientific American*. December 1983, 142–52.
A technical treatment of the aerodynamic phenomena that affect the performance of bicycles and other human-powered vehicles.

Grosser, Morton. *Gossamer Odyssey*. Boston: Houghton Mifflin Company, 1981.
The complete, official chronicle of the projects that won the Kremer prizes for human-powered flight.

Hall, William. *Cross-Country Skiing Right*. San Francisco: Harper and Row, 1985.
A guide to cross-country skiing technique.

Heese, Fred. *Canoe Racing*. Chicago: Contemporary Books, 1979.
A general treatment of canoe racing.

Howard, John. *The Cyclist's Companion*. Brattleboro, Vermont: Stephen Greene Press, 1984.
A world-class cyclist tells about the equipment, technique, and history of bicycling. Covers touring, commuting, competing, and recreational riding.

Howard, John, Albert Gross, and Christian Paul. *Multi-Fitness*. New York: Macmillan, 1985.
A cross-training system to promote fitness and health that athletes can tailor to their individual needs.

Hunt, John. *The Conquest of Everest*. New York: Dutton and Company, 1954.
The conquest of Everest by Edmund Hillary and Tenzing Norgay as described by Colonel John Hunt, the man who led the expedition.

Jacobs, Donald. *Ride and Tie*. Mountain View, California: World Publications, 1978.
A how-to book for the sport of ride and tie.

Johns, Bud. *What Is This Madness?* San Francisco: Synergistic Press, 1985.
The story of the Levi Strauss Ride and Tie as told by the man who invented the sport.

Kelly, Tom. *Birkie Fever*. Osceola, Wisconsin: Specialty Press, 1982.
History of the Birkebeiner cross-country ski race from the first race in 1973 until 1982.

Kostrubala, Thaddeus. *The Joy of Running*. Philadelphia: Lippincott, 1976.
The granddaddy of running books. Philosophical, insightful, and informative.

McDermott, Barry. "Ironman." *Sports Illustrated,* May 14, 1979, vol. 50, number 20, 88–102.
The article that inspired network-television coverage of the Ironman. Probably the seed of publicity from which mass participation in the triathlon grew.

Messner, Reinhold. (Translated by Audrey Salkeld.) *Everest*. New York: Oxford University Press, 1979.
A first-person narrative of the first assault of Everest unassisted by artificial oxygen.

Saville, Curtis and Kathleen Saville. "They Row, Row, Row Their Boat Across the Atlantic Ocean." *Smithsonian,* October 1981, 193–214.
First-person-plural account of rowing across the Atlantic.

Shermer, Michael. *Sport Cycling*. Chicago: Contemporary Books, 1985.
Marathon cycling, including everything you ever wanted to know about the Race Across AMerica.

Sillitoe, Alan. *The Loneliness of the Long-Distance Runner*. New York: Alfred Knopf, 1960.
An anthology of short stories about lower-class life in England, including a story about a long-distance runner.

Wennerberg, Conrad. *Wind, Waves and Sunburn*. New York: A. S. Barnes and Company, 1974.
A history of endurance swimming up to the mid-1970s.

PERIODICALS

Subscription addresses for selected endurance publications are given below. (Please note: magazines change their addresses and cease publication with very little warning. This list was accurate at publication, but the information for magazines can become dated fairly quickly.)

Cross Country Skiing

Cross-Country Skier
33 East Minor Street
Emmaus, Pennsylvania 18049

Cycling

Australian Cycling
163 Crown Street
East Sydney, New South Wales, 2010
Australia

Bicycle Forum
P.O. Box 8311
Missoula, Missouri 59807

Bicycle Guide
128 North 11th Street
Allentown, Pennsylvania 18102

Bicycle Rider
29901 Agoura Road
Agoura, California 91301

Bicycle USA
P.O. Box 988
Baltimore, Maryland 21203

Bicycling
33 East Minor Street
Emmaus, Pennsylvania 18049

Bicycling News Canada
101–1281 West Georgia Street
Vancouver, British Columbia
V6E 3J7
Canada

Cycling
Currey House 1 Thrawley Way
Sutton, Surrey SMa 4QQ
England

Cyclist
P.O. Box 993
Farmingdale, New York 11737–0001

Human Power
International Human-Powered
  Vehicle Association
P.O. Box 2068
Seal Beach, California 90740

Southwest Cycling
11684 Ventura Boulevard
Number 213
Studio City, California 91604

Velo-News
P.O. Box 1257
Brattleboro, Vermont 05301

Winning: Bicycle Racing Illustrated
1524 Linden Street
Allentown, Pennsylvania 18102

Endurance Horseback Riding
Endurance News
701 High Street
Suite 216
Auburn, California 95603

Trail Blazer
P.O. Box 1855
Paso Robles, California 93446

Endurance Sports in General
City Sports
P.O. Box 3693
San Francisco, California 94119

Outside
1165 North Clark Street
Chicago, Illinois 60610

Sportswise
1633 Broadway
New York, New York 10019

Superfit
33 East Minor Street
Emmaus, Pennsylvania 18049

Ultrasport
P.O. Box 27938
San Diego, California 92127

Wisconsin Silent Sports
P.O. Box 152
Waupaca, Wisconsin 54981

Women's Sports
P.O. Box 612
Holmes, Pennsylvania 19043

Rowing and Paddling
The American Canoeist
American Canoe Association
Box 248
Lorton, Virginia 22079

American Whitewater Association Journal
American Whitewater Affiliation
Box 1483
Hagerstown, Maryland 21740

Canoe
P.O. Box 10748
Des Moines, Iowa 50347–0748

Canoe News
United States Canoe Association
P.O. Box 5743
Lafayette, Indiana 47904

Currents
National Organization for River
  Sports
P.O. Box 6847
Colorado Springs, Colorado 80934

River Runner
Box 2047
Vista, California 92083

Rowing USA
U.S. Rowing Association
251 North Illinois Street
Suite 980
Indianapolis, Indiana 46204

Sea Kayaker
1670 Duranleau Street
Vancouver, British Columbia
V6H 3S4
Canada

Running

Arizona Running News
4609 East Thomas Road
Phoenix, Arizona 85018

Inside Running
8100 Bellair Boulevard
Number 1318
Houston, Texas 77036

Joe Henderson's Running Com-
  mentator
4620 Manzanita Street
Eugene, Oregon 97405

Northwest Runner
1231 North East 94th Street
Seattle, Washington 98115

Racing South
P.O. Box 448
Stone Mountain, Georgia 30086

The Runner
P.O. Box 2730
Boulder, Colorado 80322

Running News
New York Road Runners Club
9 East 89th Street
New York, New York 10128

Running Times
14416 Jefferson Davis Highway
Suite 20
Woodbridge, Virginia 22191

Runner's World
33 East Minor Street
Emmaus, Pennsylvania 18049

Ultrarunning
P.O. Box 1057
Amherst, Massachusetts 01004

Swimming

Ocean Sports International
10 Seacliff Drive
Number 10
Aptos, California

Swim
P.O. Box 2168
Simi Valley, California 93062

Swimming World
P.O. Box 45497
Los Angeles, California 90045

Triathlon

Australian Triathlon Sports
P.O. Box 1014
Bondi Junction, 202, Sydney
Australia

New Zealand Triathlete
P.O. Box 55–042
Auckland, New Zealand

Running and Triathlon News
5111 Santa Fe Street
San Diego, California 92109

Triathlete
8461 Warner Drive
Culver City, California 90232

Tri-Fit Quarterly
575 Burns Street
Penticton, British Columbia
V2A 4W9
Canada

(*Triathlete* is the magazine that was created when *Tri-Athlete* and *Triathlon* merged in 1986.)